S0-ASK-222

EKG Technician Program
Standard Student Workbook

Fourth Custom Edition for
Condensed Curriculum International

Taken from:
EKG: Plain and Simple: PowerPoint Lecture
by Karen Ellis

Cover Art: Courtesy of Chaikom, PeterPhoto123/Shutterstock

Excerpts taken from:

EKG: Plain and Simple: PowerPoint Lecture
by Karen Ellis
Copyright © 2017, 2012, 2007 by Pearson Education, Inc.
New York, NY 10013

Pearson Education, Inc., 330 Hudson Street, New York, New York 10013
A Pearson Education Company
www.pearsoned.com

Printed in the United States of America

4   2019

000200010272192656

EF

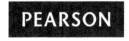
ISBN 10: 0-135-73810-5
ISBN 13: 978-0-135-73810-8

TABLE OF CONTENTS

PART A
EKG Technician

STUDENT PACKET INFORMATION

TABLE OF CONTENTS

The EKG Technician Program

COURSE DESCRIPTION

The EKG technician is an integral part of the cardiology diagnostic team, frequently performing the initial testing that assists the physician in identifying abnormal cardiac arrhythmias.

The EKG technician program instructs the students on the technical and clinical aspects of EKG performance. Attention is given to quality, accuracy and safety throughout the program with a focus on not only understanding the proper lead placement for the 12 lead EKG but also a rudimentary knowledge of basic cardiac arrhythmias. Students also perform hands on EKGs and are eligible to sit for a National EKG Certification Exam upon the successful completion of the program.

EXPECTATIONS FOR THE STUDENT

1. Students are expected to arrive for class on time

2. Absent students must contact their instructor prior to class time

3. Absent students will be expected to make up missed class work/assignments on their own time

4. Students will follow the rules and regulations of the facility

5. No student shall disrupt a class or interfere with the session or the learning or the other students

6. The Instructor will be the student's contact for all academic questions or concerns

7. Cell phones and pagers are to be turned off or to the vibrator mode while in class

8. Any student participating in any act of academic dishonesty, such as cheating, plagiarism, or collusion will be considered for dismissal from the program. Once dismissed, no condition of re-entrance will be considered.

EKG EXAMINATION INFORMATION

The following outlines the subject matter covered in the EKG Examination and throughout this course:

I. The Heart

- terminology related to the heart
- the anatomy and physiology of the heart and its function
- the cardiac cycle as well as the structure and function of each part
- the coronary blood supply and the specifics of a myocardium infarct
- common disorders and diseases of the heart
- blood pressure and related vital signs

II. The Conduction System

- definitions and terminology related to the conduction system
- conduction system, its parts, locations, and functions
- the order of impulse
- conduction impulses related to the pumping mechanism

III. The Electrocardiogram

- terminology related to the EKG machine
- the function of the EKG in diagnosis and treatment
- the EKG machine and its related parts
- the cardiac cycle as it is displayed on the EKG tracing
- the P-Q-R-S-T segments and waves including their meaning and appearance
- the EKG paper, its parts and how measurements are established
- EKG lead placement, what each lead measures, and how they are marked and recorded
- proper patient preparation
- recognize common artifact and other arrhythmia

EKG CERTIFICATION EXAM

Students that successfully complete this course are eligible to sit for certain EKG Certification exams. During this course the instructor will receive an application for each student to complete for the certification exam. The students will be instructed to take the information home to review and complete independently. An examination date will be established by CCI and the instructor. Once this date has been established the date will be given to the students.

All applications and the required funds must be submitted 30 days prior to this exam date. Students must successfully complete the following eligibility requirements to sit for the exam:

- Successfully complete the EKG course
- Perform a minimum of 5 mounted EKGs
- Submit one mounted EKG with the completed examination signed by both the student and the instructor
- Submit a letter from the instructor stating the successful completion of all requirements

TEACHING METHODS EMPLOYED

Lecture, class discussion, group discussions, role-playing, critical thinking exercises, and application activities related to EKG. This course also includes hands on instruction in obtaining an EKG.

EVALUATION AND GRADE DETERMINATION

Student performance will be evaluated utilizing the following analysis:

- Attendance and class participation (50%)
- Quizzes (25%)
- Final Exam (25%)

It is vital that each student recognize that this class is a pass/fail class.

SYLLABUS

The attached syllabus provides a class-by-class outline of the materials to be discussed during class as well as the homework assigned for the following class. This syllabus is a guideline and may be adjusted to the needs of the class at the discretion of the instructor.

EKG TECHNICIAN
SYLLABUS

Instructor: _____

Contact: Phone _____

                             E-Mail_____

Class Time: _____

Required Textbook:

1. <u>EKG Technician Program: Standard; Second Custom Edition for Condensed Curriculum International</u>

2. <u>EKG Technician Program: Standard Student Workbook; Third Custom Edition for Condensed Curriculum International</u>

The course outline attached will indicate the information that will be covered in each class and what homework assignments will be required for the next class. This syllabus is subject to revision based on the needs of the class.

The students are responsible for the following:

- All homework assignments and preparation is to be completed prior to class.
- Students are responsible for all homework assignments, schedules quizzes/tests, and hands-on experience (if applicable). If any of these is missed due to absenteeism or tardiness, the student is responsible to make up the missed work to successfully complete this course.
- The above instructor contact information is to be used in the event of anticipated student absenteeism.
- Student effort and commitment is necessary to understanding the course materials. It is <u>strongly recommended</u> that all course materials be reviewed and studied prior to and following each class.

PART B
EKG Technician Program

STUDENT HANDOUTS AND STUDY GUIDE

TABLE OF CONTENTS

The following pages have been developed to provide a summary of the materials to be studied in preparation for the EKG Certification Exam. These materials in no way represent all the knowledge required to successfully complete this course or the certification exam. All materials and class discussion are to be utilized for these achievements. It is vital that to successfully challenge the certification exam, the student must study all materials presented by the instructor throughout this course.

Chapter 1

The EKG
Technician Program
Student Handout #1

ANATOMY AND PHYSIOLOGY OF THE CARDIOVASCULAR SYSTEM

- The cardiovascular system is composed of the heart and blood vessels.
- The heart is the organ that moves blood through the circulatory system and thus to and from each part of the body.
- It is located in the mediastinum cavity. It is a hollow organ that works as a pump.
- The top of the heart (called the base) lies just below the second rib.
- The apex or bottom of the heart is at a point between the fifth and sixth ribs and points to the left.
- The heart has four chambers. The two upper chambers are called the atria. The two lower chambers are called the ventricles.
- The right and left sides are divided by the septum with the two atria divided by the interatrial septum and the two ventricles divided by the interventricular septum.
- The right heart pumps blood into the pulmonary circulatory system (the blood vessels within the lungs and those carrying blood to and from the lungs).
- The left heart pumps blood into the systemic circulatory system (the blood vessels in the rest of the body and those carrying blood to and from the body).
- Heart performs its pumping action over and over in rhythmic sequence.
- The period of relaxation and filling of the ventricles with blood is diastole.
- The period during which the ventricles contract and empty blood is systole.
- The pumping action of the heart is referred to as the mechanical response.
- The heart wall is made up of three separate and distinct layers:
  - The outer layer is called the epicardium.
  - The middle layer is called the myocardium. The myocardium is made up of layers and bands of cardiac muscle fiber with complex spirals.
  - The inner layer, the endocardium. The endocardium is a thin membrane that lines the chambers of the heart, covers the valves, and is continuous with the lining of the major blood vessels that enter the heart.
  - The heart is enclosed in the pericardium, a tough but loose fitting sac that covers and protects the heart.

- There are four valves located within the heart with the AV valves held in place by the chordea tendinea:
  - The pulmonary semilunar valve prevents the back flow of blood into the right ventricle as it leaves by way of the pulmonary artery.
  - The aortic semilunar valve prevents the back flow of blood from the aorta into the left ventricle.
  - The valve between the right atrium and the right ventricle is called the tricuspid valve. It has three flaps or cusps, thus the name tricuspid.
  - The valve between the left ventricle and the left atrium is the bicuspid or mitral valve. These two valves are called the atrioventricular valves (AV valves).
- Blood carrying carbon dioxide returns from the body below the diaphragm by way of the inferior vena cava and from the body above the diaphragm through the superior vena cava where it enters into the right atrium.
- When the right atrium contracts the blood is forced through the tricuspid valve into the right ventricle.
- When the right ventricle contracts the blood is pushed through the pulmonary semilunar valve to the right and left pulmonary arteries, which are the only arteries that carry carbon dioxide laden blood. From these arteries blood travels into the lungs.
- In the lungs, carbon dioxide is given off, and the blood is replenished with oxygen.
- The left and right pulmonary veins, which are the only veins that carry oxygenated blood, allow the oxygenated blood from the lungs to return to the left atrium of the heart.
- As the left atrium contracts it forces the blood through the mitral (bicuspid) valve into the left ventricle.
- The left ventricle is the largest chamber of the heart. When it contracts, it forces the oxygenated blood through the aortic semilunar valve into the aorta to be distributed throughout the body.

Arteries and Veins

- Blood is transported to every part of the body by the action of the heart as it pumps the blood through the network of the vascular system of arteries and veins.
- The arteries leaving the heart are the largest. They branch into smaller arteries and finally even smaller vessels called arterioles. These continue to branch into the capillaries.
- Once the exchange of oxygen and carbon dioxide (and other nutrients and gasses) occurs in the capillary bed, the blood flows into the small vessels called venules and then into the veins.
- The veins return the blood to the heart. They also branch into the capillaries. Thus, the cardiovascular system is a closed system.
- The heart pumps the blood through the arteries and arterioles to the capillaries; in the capillaries, the exchange of carbon dioxide and oxygen takes place. The deoxygenated blood then enters into the venules, and then to the veins through which the blood returns to the heart.
- There are two major circuits that are formed by the blood vessels. These are called the pulmonary and the systemic:

  1. **Pulmonary Circuit** The pulmonary arteries carry blood containing carbon dioxide from the heart to the lungs. Oxygenated blood from the lungs is then returned to the heart by the pulmonary veins. This is the only time in the body in which an artery carries deoxygenated blood and a vein carries oxygenated blood.
  2. **Systemic Circulation** Made up of all other arteries and veins. These vessels carry oxygen and nutrients to all tissues of the body and then transport the wastes for disposal from all tissues except the lungs.

Coronary Arteries

- Blood is supplied to the myocardium during the diastole phase by two main arteries called the R & L coronary arteries
- RCA – supplies blood to the Rt Atrium, Rt ventricle, inferior surface and posterior walls of the Lt ventricle, AV node 90%, SA node 55%, and proximal portion of the bundle of His
- LCA divides into two branches – **LAD** – Feeds the anterior surface of the Lt ventricle, all bundle branches and part of the Rt ventricle – **Circumflex** – feeds the Lt Atrium, lateral wall of the heart and the SA node 45% and the AV node 10%
- Additional circulation exists when existing coronary arteries become blocked and collateral circulation will form

LOCATION OF THE HEART

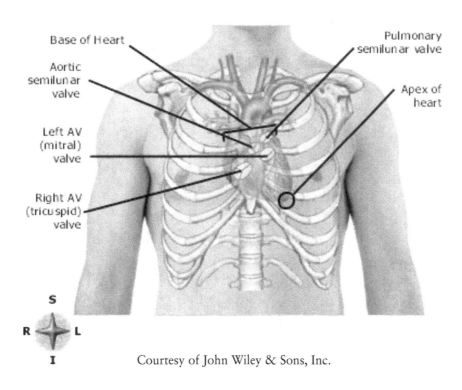

Courtesy of John Wiley & Sons, Inc.

ANATOMY OF THE HEART

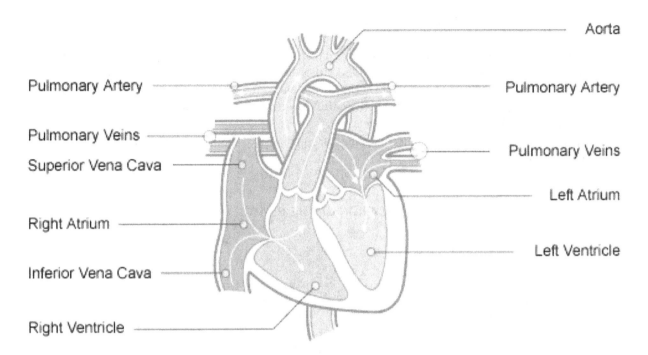

Chapter 2.

The EKG Technician Program
Student Handout #2

CONDUCTION SYSTEM

- In most cases, in order for the heart to pump (mechanical response) it receives an electrical stimulus. This electrical stimulus comes from the electrical system.
- Specialized electrical cells called pacemaker cells in the heart are arranged in a system of pathways called the conductions system
- It is composed of the following structures: SA node, Internodal tract, AV junction consisting of the AV node and Bundle of His, RBBB, LBBB and purkinje network
- The primary function of the conduction system is to transmit minute electrical impulses from the SA node to the atria and ventricles, causing them to contract
- With normal conduction, impulses originate in the SA node (pacemaker), travel down to the AV node through the bundle of His and down the purkinje fibers
- Normally the pacemaker site with the fastest rate controls the heart
- In normal conduction, the dominant pacemaker is the SA node with an inherent rate of 60 to 100 bpm
- The AV junction, bundle branches, and purkinje fibers can all act as escape pacemakers when the SA node fails
- Escape – a term used when the sinus node slows down or fails to initiate depolarization and the lower site becomes the pacemaker
- The inherent rate for the AV junction is 40 to 60 bpm
- The inherent rate for the bundle branches and purkinje network is 20–40 bpm
- Premature beats refers to beats that occur as a result of irritability. It is possible for a new site to take over as the pacemaker because that site is either generating an impulse or impulses faster than the normal pacemaker

The structures that make up the heart's conduction system:

1. **Sinoatrial or SA Node**
   - A cluster of cells located in the upper wall of the right atrium
   - Normally depolarizes faster than any other part of the conduction system, that is why it is the heart's normal pacemaker

- Other areas can take over by discharging impulses more rapidly than the SA node or by passively taking over when the SA node has failed or is generating impulses too slowly
- Fires at a rate of 60 to 100 beats per minute (bpm)
- Once the impulse leaves the SA node it causes depolarization of the adjacent myocardial cells resulting in their contraction. The impulse continues to spread from cell to cell in a wavelike form across the atrial muscle causing atrial contraction
- Seen on the EKG monitor as a P wave

2. **Atrioventricular or AV Node**
   - Specialized cells located in the lower portion of the atrium above the base of the tricuspid valve
   - Has no pacemaker cells itself, surrounding area does
   - Has 2 functions, delays electrical impulses in order to allow the atria to contract and complete filling of the ventricles before the next contraction and it receives an electrical impulse which it conducts to the ventricles

3. **Bundle of His**
   - Receives impulses from the AV node, is located in the upper portion of the interventricular septum and connects the AV node to the 2 bundle branches
   - Has pacemaking cells capable of firing at an intrinsic rate of 40–60 bpm
   - AV node and Bundle of His are referred to as the AV Junction

4. **Right and Left Bundle Branches**
   - Responsible for ventricular contraction represented by the QRS complex
   - Comprised of the Rt and Lt Bundle Branches
   - LBB divides into 2 bundles called fascicles to supply the Lt ventricle which is thicker and more muscular
   - The purkinje fibers are an elaborate web of fibers that penetrate 1/3 of the way into the ventricles
   - The intrinsic rate is <40 bpm

CARDIAC CELLS

There are two types of cells in the heart:

- Myocardial cells- found in the myocardium, responsible for contraction and relaxation, have property of contractility. Electrically stimulated contractile filaments that slide together causing contraction
- Specialized cells of electrical conduction – found in conduction system responsible for the generation and conduction of electrical impulses. These cells have a property of automaticity and conductivity. No contractile filaments, spontaneous generation and conduction of electrical impulses (pacemaker cells)

Four Primary Characteristics of Cardiac Cells

- Excitability – or irritability shared by all cardiac cells. Refers to the ability of the cardiac muscle cells to respond to an outside stimuli
- Automaticity – ability of cardiac pacemaker cells to spontaneously initiate an electrical impulse without being stimulated from another source

- Conductivity – ability of a cardiac cell to receive an electrical stimulus and conduct that impulse to an adjacent cardiac cell
- Contractility – ability of cardiac cells to shorten causing contraction in response to an electrical stimuli

Nervous Control of the Heart

- The heart rate is controlled by both the sympathetic and parasympathetic nervous systems
- The medulla in the brain contains 2 cardiac centers: Accelerator Center and the Inhibitory Center
- Stimulation of the sympathetic nerve fibers results in the release of norepinephrine, which increases the force of ventricular contractions, heart rate, blood pressure and CO
- The sympathetic nerve fibers controls both the atria and the ventricles but primarily the ventricles
- Stimulation of the parasympathetic nerve fibers comes from the inhibitory center of the medulla via the vagus nerve
- Stimulation of these nerve fibers can cause the release of acetylcholine, which results in the slowing of the heart rate

Depolarization and Repolarization

- Before the heart can mechanically contract and pump blood, cardiac muscle cell depolarization must take place
- A difference between electrical charges must exist in order for an electrical current to be generated
- Major electrolytes that affect cardiac function are sodium (Na+), Potassium (K+) and Calcium (CA+)
- The exchange of electrolytes in myocardial cells creates electrical activity which appears on the EKG as waveforms
- Depolarization and Repolarization occur in a five phase cycle – Action potential, which is a reflection of the difference in the concentration of the these ions across the cell membrane
- Depolarization occurs as a result of the movement of ions across the cell membrane
- Depolarization is not the same as contraction. Contraction is a result of depolarization

Absolute/Relative Refractory Periods

- Absolute – This period occurs at the onset of the QRS to the peak of the T wave. During this period, myocardial cells do not contract and cells conduction system will not conduct
- Relative Refractory – This period occurs during the down slope of the T wave. During this period, some cardiac cells have repolarized to their threshold potential and can be stimulated to depolarize if the stimulus is strong enough

CONDUCTION SYSTEM

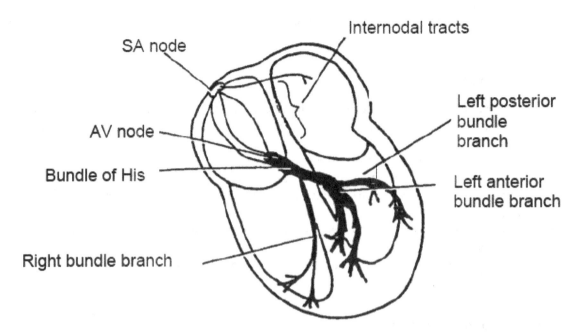

Courtesy of Twin Cities Health Professional Education Consortium

The EKG
Technician Program
Student Handout #3

12-Lead EKG Placement

To obtain an ECG the patient must be supine on a comfortable bed or exam table. Ten electrodes must be placed at precise anatomical locations on the patient to obtain optimal quality data. Remember, before any lead can be placed, the electrode area of the patient's skin should be cleaned with alcohol (and gauze) to remove oil, sweat, or scaly skin. Failure to apply the electrodes to a clean surface could result in baseline drift. The patient must have loose clothing and be free of excessive body hair. For a male patient with excessive hair, the points at which the leads are connected must be shaved. Female patients must remove upper undergarments to allow for lead placement. It is also best to instruct the patient not to use lotion on the day of the ECG.

Limb Leads

Start with the right leg. The right leg electrode is to be applied to the inner leg about 4–5 cm. above the ankle. Prepare the skin with alcohol and gauze and rub the area vigorously about ten times. Peel an electrode from the carrier card and apply to the skin, pressing gently to ensure good adhesion. Parting the hair during applications helps adhesion. The tab end of the electrode is pointed toward the upper leg. Follow the same procedure to apply the left leg electrode. Next, go to the right arm. The inside of the lower arm has thinner skin and is the preferred electrode site. Prepare the skin with alcohol and gauze and rub the area vigorously about ten times. Place the electrode on the right arm so that the tab of the electrode is pointing up towards the arm. Follow the same procedures to apply the left arm electrode.

Attach the lead wires to the four extremities. Select the correct wire from the patient cable distribution block and pull it from the group. Attach the clip into the electrode. The cable lead wires need to be as straight as possible. Loops in the lead wires can cause interference. One limb lead should be placed on each arm and one on each leg. The position on the extremities is not crucial but should be consistent and placed on an area devoid of excessive hair. Care should be taken to be sure the left and right arm leads (aVR, aVL, lead I) are placed correctly. Reversal of the arm leads is the most common error in lead placement.

According to the American Heart Association, "The electrodes may be placed on any part of the arms or of the legs as long as they are below the shoulders in the former and below the inguinal fold anteriorly and the gluteal fold posteriorly in the latter. Any other placement necessary by deformed or missing extremities must be noted on the record."

LL left leg (by ankle)

LA left forearm

RA right forearm

RL right leg (by ankle)

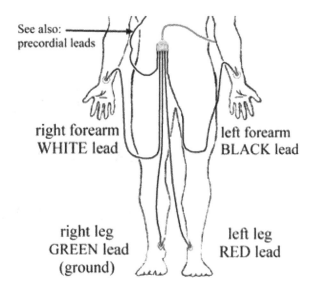

See also: precordial leads

right forearm
WHITE lead

left forearm
BLACK lead

right leg
GREEN lead
(ground)

left leg
RED lead

Chest Leads

The placement of the precordial electrode is often too casual. The placement should be as exact and constant as possible. For this reason only bony landmarks should be used in locating the precordial points. Even small displacements of the electrodes may produce considerable changes in the pattern.

Palpate the patient's chest to locate the appropriate sites for the precordial leads. Locate the sternal angle with two fingers and move fingers towards the patient's right side to palpate the 1st and 2nd intercostal space. Keep moving down the intercostal spaces until the 4th intercostal space at the right border of the sternum is located.

Place each of the chest leads in the following way:

1. V1 4th intercostal space, right of sternum

2. V2 4th intercostal space, left of sternum

3. V3 midway between V2 and V4

4. V4 5th intercostal space, in the midclavicular line

5. V5 same level as V4, at anterior axillary line (between V4 and V6)

6. V6 in 5th intercostal space, in the midaxillary line

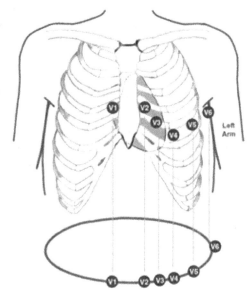

Courtesy of drbloggs.com

Recording Quality Electrocardiograms

It is extremely important that the electrocardiograms submitted have a clean baseline, are free of drift, muscle tremor, and A-C interference. Enough variables influence the tracing without introducing unnecessary technical ones. It is the responsibility of the technician to produce high quality ECG's, using uniform techniques from tracing to tracing every day. Some of the most frequently found problems are discussed in this section.

- **Baseline Drift or Baseline Wander** – Baseline drift is probably the most frequently encountered problem in the ECG. Check each of the leads for good contact. Clean or shave any area as required.
- **Muscle Tremor Interference** – Muscle tremor is an artifact signal which is usually generated by the arm and leg muscles. These signals are present when the patient is tense, cold, or affected with muscle or nerve disorders. Reassure and try to relax the patient. Limb leads can be placed on the upper arms and thighs to eliminate muscle tremor caused by the arms and legs. (This in no way affects the accuracy of the ECG), or place a pillow under the patient's knees to slightly elevate the legs.
- **A-C Interference** – A-C interference is a common problem in a clinic or hospital setting. It can be caused by poor electrode contact or interference from nearby equipment. Keep all unused equipment away from the exam area.
- **Electrodes Falling Off** – Electrodes on hairy chests and loose skin can be a problem and certain precautions can save time in connecting a patient. To help with this problem, try the following: establish a good connection by parting the hair before attaching the electrode, if the wire is twisted, it may tend to pull at the electrode

WANDERING BASELINE

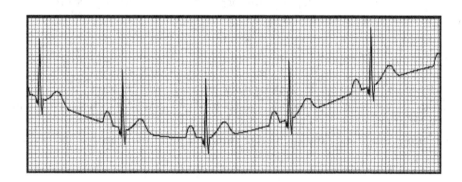

The EKG Technician Program
Student Handout #4

Blood Pressure

- Blood pressure is the amount of force placed on the artery walls during cardiac contraction and relaxation
- The normal BP is 120/80
- The top number, called the systolic #, represents the amount of force placed on the arteries when the heart is beating
- The bottom number, called the diastolic #, represents the amount of pressure felt on the arteries when the heart is at rest or in between beats

ECG Paper

- The horizontal axis measures amplitude and the vertical axis measures time
- Each small square measures .04 seconds and each large square containing five small squares represents .20 seconds
- Each square represents 1 mm and each large square containing 5 small squares represents 5 mm

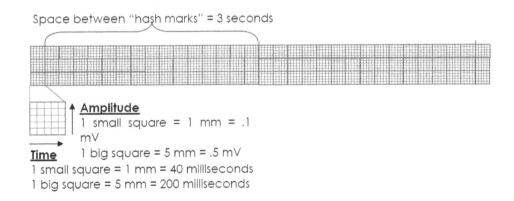

Space between "hash marks" = 3 seconds

Amplitude
1 small square = 1 mm = .1 mV
1 big square = 5 mm = .5 mV

Time
1 small square = 1 mm = 40 milliseconds
1 big square = 5 mm = 200 milliseconds

Standardized Mark on the ECG Tracing

The standardized mark (Π) is at the beginning of each line on the ECG tracing. This mark represents the standard amplitude that the ECG machine measures. This rate is 10 mm or two large blocks in height. Today, most machines are computerized and the machine completes the standardization automatically. In a manual machine, the standardization must be established in the following way prior to every ECG:

- When the strip is running, depress the St'D button to place the amplitude mark
- Ensure that the mark is the equivalent of 2 large blocks or 10 mm in height

Evaluating the Waves

In NSR each wave of the ECG is identified by a letter and represents an action within the heart

- P wave   Represents the contraction/depolarization/systole of the atria
- PR Interval   Represents the time it takes for the impulse to travel from the SA node to the Bundle of His
- QRS complex   Represents the contraction/depolarization/systole of the ventricles
- T wave   Represents the relaxation/repolarization/diastole of the ventricles
- U wave   Represents an abnormally low potassium
- Isoelectric   Represents no electrical activity or a balance at the cellular level called polarization

Evaluating the P wave (represents the contraction (systole) of the atria in NSR)

The P wave has a characteristic shape that will often stick out among a lot of unidentifiable waves. It is usually rounded, upright, and uniform.
    When examining the rhythm strip for P waves ask yourself the following questions:

- Is there one P wave for every QRS?
- Are the P waves regular?
- Is the P wave in front of the QRS or behind it?
- Is the P wave normal and upright in Lead II?
- Are there more P waves than QRS complexes?
- Do all the P waves look alike?

Determining the PRI

The PR interval represents the time it takes for the electrical impulse to travel from the SA node to the bundle of His. Normally it should take anywhere from 0.12 to 0.20 seconds and is measured from the beginning of the P wave to the beginning of the QRS complex. When measuring the PR interval do the following:

- Count the number of small squares between the start of the P wave to the start of QRS complex and multiply the number by 0.04.
- Ask yourself; is the duration normal (0.12 to 0.20 seconds)?
- Is the PR interval constant?

Determining the Duration of the QRS Complex (represents the contraction (systole) of the ventricles)

The QRS duration represents the spread of the impulse through the ventricular muscle, or what is called ventricular depolarization. Determine the QRS complex through the following steps:

- Measure straight across the front end of the PR interval to the end of the S wave, not just the peak.
- To calculate the duration, count the number of small squares between the beginning and end of the QRS complex and multiply by 0.04 seconds
- Is the duration normal (less than .12 seconds)?
- Are all the QRS complexes the same size and shape?
- Does a QRS complex appear after every P wave?

To interpret arrhythmias you must be able to measure the PR interval and the duration of the QRS complex. Grid markings on the graph paper are used to determine just how many seconds it took for the impulse to create those intervals.

The ST Segment

The ST segment represents the resting period between depolarization and repolarization in NSR. Normally it is seen as a flat isoelectric line and begins at the beginning of the S to the beginning of the T wave. A normal ST segment has the following characteristics:

- Usually isoelectric (neither positive or negative) and may vary from –0.5 to +1 mm in some pre-cordial leads

The T Wave

The T wave represents ventricular recovery or repolarization. When evaluating a normal T wave, determine the following:

- Follows the S wave
- Amplitude is 0.5 mm in leads I, II, and III and up to 10 mm in the precordial leads
- The configuration is typically round and smooth
- The deflection is usually the same as the QRS complex (typically a positive deflection)

The QT Interval

The QT interval measures ventricular depolarization and repolarization. An abnormality in duration may indicate myocardial or possible sclerotic problems. A normal QT interval has the following characteristics:

- Location – extends from the beginning of the QRS complex to the end of the T wave
- Duration varies according to age, sex, and heart rate and usually lasts from 0.36 to 0.44 seconds

WAVEFORM DURING A NORMAL SINUS RHYTHM

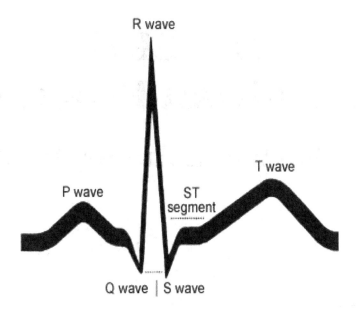

The EKG
Technician Program
Student Handout #5

THE EKG TECHNICIAN

Electrocardiograph (EKG or ECG) Technicians operate equipment that records and measures heart activity. These measurements are used to assist cardiologists and other physicians in diagnosing and treating cardiac (heart) and peripheral vascular (blood vessel) problems. An EKG technician first obtains a patient's medical history and medication use. Then they prepare a patient by attaching electrodes to the chest, arms, and legs. These electrodes will measure trace electrical impulses transmitted by the heart in order to obtain a printout that can be used by the physician. These tests are often done as part of routine examination before surgeries, especially on older patients or those that have a history of cardiovascular problems. With additional on-the-job training or experience, EKG technicians may specialize in areas such as cardiac catheterization, Holter monitoring, phonocardiography, stress testing, and vectorcardiography. EKG technicians must be able to recognize an emergency and assist the physician in responding to them.

The EKG technician must be organized, efficient, flexible, and multifunctional with the ability to work independently. Good initiative and communication skills, as well as good public relation skills are important when working with patients, co-workers, desk attendants and supervisors.

PATIENT PREPARATION FOR ELECTROCARDIOGRAMS

Communication

Although all of us have been communicating with others since our infancy, the process of transmitting information from an individual (or group) to another is a very complex process with many sources of potential error.

In any communication at least some of the "meaning" is lost in simple transmission of a message from the sender to the receiver. In many situations a lot of the true message is lost and the message that is heard is often far different than the one intended. This is most obvious in cross-cultural situations where language is an issue. But it is also common among people of the same culture.

It is also very important to understand that a majority of communication is non-verbal. This means that when we attribute meaning to what someone else is saying, the verbal part of the message actually means less than the non-verbal part. The non-verbal part includes such things as a clinched jaw, rolling of eyes and slumped posture.

Skill in communication involves a number of specific strengths. The first we will discuss involves listening skills. The following lists some suggestions for effective listening

- Listen openly and with empathy to the other person
- Judge the content, not the messenger or delivery; comprehend before you judge
- Use multiple techniques to fully comprehend (ask, repeat, rephrase, etc.)
- Active body state; fight distractions
- Ask the other person for as much detail as he/she can provide; paraphrase what the other is saying to make sure you understand it and check for understanding
- Respond in an interested way that shows you understand the communication
- Attend to non-verbal cues, body language, not just words; listen between the lines
- Ask the other for his views or suggestions
- Be descriptive, not evaluative-describe objectively, your reactions, consequences
- Be validating, not invalidating ("You wouldn't understand"); acknowledge other's uniqueness, importance
- Be conjunctive, not disjunctive (not "I want to discuss this regardless of what you want to discuss")
- Don't totally control conversation; acknowledge what was said
- Own up: use "I", not "They" . . . not "I've heard you are noncooperative"
- Don't react to emotional words, but interpret their purpose
- Practice supportive listening, not one way listening

In addition, a supportive and effective listener does the following:

- Stop Talking: Asks the other person for as much detail as he/she can provide; asks for other's views and suggestions
- Looks at the person, listens openly and with empathy to the employee; is clear about his position; be patient
- Listen and Respond in an interested way that shows you understand the problem and the other's concern
- Is validating, not invalidating ("You wouldn't understand"); acknowledge other's uniqueness, importance
- Checks for understanding; paraphrases; asks questions for clarification
- Don't control conversation; acknowledge what was said; let the other finish before responding
- Focuses on the problem, not the person; is descriptive and specific, not evaluative; focuses on content, not delivery or emotion
- React to the message, not the person, delivery or emotion
- Make sure you comprehend before you judge; ask questions
- Use many techniques to fully comprehend
- Stay in an active body state to aid listening
- Fight distractions
- Avoid using medical terms that the patient may not understand

DEALING WITH LEGAL ASPECTS AND ETHICS IN HEALTH CARE

Professionalism and Attitude

Being an ECG technician not only requires skill and training, but also that you possess both enthusiasm and a concerned and positive attitude. Professionalism involves those characteristics and personal traits that make up an individual who is committed to performing his or her job in an accurate and efficient manner.

Because medicine is a *profession* and EKG technicians are *professionals*, it is important to have a clear understanding of what "professionalism" means. As an EKG technician-in-training, you will be developing a personal sense of what it means to be a professional.

What Does It Mean To Be a Member of a Profession?

The words "profession" and "professional" come from the Latin word "professio," which means a public declaration with the force of a promise. Professions are groups which declare in a public way that their members promise to perform in certain ways and that the group and the society may discipline those who fail to do so. The profession presents itself to society as a social benefit and society accepts the profession, expecting it to serve some important social goal. The profession usually issues a code of ethics stating the standards by which its members can be judged. The traditional professions are medicine, law, education and clergy.

The marks of a profession are:

1. Competence in a specialized body of knowledge and skill;

2. An acknowledgment of specific duties and responsibilities toward the individuals it serves and toward society;

3. The right to train, admit, discipline and dismiss its members for failure to sustain competence or observe the duties and responsibilities.

What Is the Difference between a Profession and a Business?

The line between a business and a profession is not entirely clear, since professionals may engage in business and make a living by it. However, one crucial difference distinguishes them: professionals have a *fiduciary duty* toward those they serve. This means that professionals have a particularly stringent duty to assure that their decisions and actions serve the welfare of their patients, even at some cost to themselves. Professions have codes of ethics which specify the obligations arising from this fiduciary duty. Ethical problems often occur when there appears to be a conflict between these obligations or between fiduciary duties and personal goals.

What Are the Recognized Obligations and Values of a Professional EKG Technician?

Professionalism requires that the technician strive for excellence in the following areas which should be modeled by mentors and teachers and become part of the attitudes, behaviors, and skills integral to patient care:

- Altruism: A technician is obligated to attend to the best interest of patients, rather than self-interest.
- Accountability: EKG technicians are accountable to their patients, to society on issues of public health, and to their profession.
- Excellence: EKG technicians are obligated to make a commitment to life-long learning.
- Duty: A technician should be available and responsive when "on call," accepting a commitment to service within the profession and the community.
- Honor and integrity: EKG technicians should be committed to being fair, truthful and straight-forward in their interactions with patients and the profession.
- Respect for others: A technician should demonstrate respect for patients and their families, other EKG technicians and team members.

These values should provide guidance for promoting professional behavior and for making difficult ethical decisions.

PATIENT CONSENT

Levels of Consent

As with any medical procedure, we need the patient's consent to perform an EKG. The decision to undergo a medical procedure rests with the patient who, if competent, retains the right to exercise control over his or her body. Consent may be given by the patient, or by someone authorized to give consent on behalf of the patient. There are two levels of consent — basic consent and informed consent.

Basic consent: The EKG Technician must have permission to touch the patient. Often, basic consent is implied. For example, if the patient comes to the clinic or hospital for the EKG, the patient's consent for the test is implied. Likewise, if the patient puts on a gown in the physician's office in preparation for the EKG, the patient is impliedly giving consent to the EKG technician to perform the test. Failure to obtain basic consent exposes the technician to a claim of medical battery. Two questions must be asked to determine whether the technician/facility may be liable for medical battery. Was the patient aware that the technician was going to perform the procedure? If so, did the patient authorize the procedure? If the answer to either of these questions is "no," the patient has a claim for medical battery.

Informed consent: Although an informed consent is typically not required for an EKG, it may be required for a more high–risk diagnostic cardiac test such as stress test. Before a patient can make an informed decision about what medical care to accept or reject, the patient must have adequate information. Medical professionals have a duty before performing a procedure to provide an adequate explanation to assist the patient's decision-making process. Generally, informed consent should include pertinent information about:

- The diagnosis and nature of the patient's problem;
- The purpose of the proposed treatment and its benefits;
- Any material risks of the proposed treatment;
- The risks and benefits of reasonable alternative treatments;
- The prognosis if the proposed treatment is refused; and
- Whether the proposed treatment is experimental.

LEGAL TERMS

- **Advance Directive** – An individual instruction or a written statement relating to the subsequent provision of health care for the individual, including, but not limited to a living will or a durable power of attorney for health care.
- **Beneficence** – Creates an obligation to benefit patients and other persons and to further their welfare and interests.
- **Emancipated Minor** – A minor who is financially independent and who is no longer under the control or authority of his or her parents or guardian (this may be evidenced by a court order), a married minor, or a minor in the armed services.
- **General Consent** – The type of consent that must be obtained before touching the patient.
- **Guardian** – A judicially appointed guardian or conservator having authority to make a health care decision for an individual.
- **Informed Consent** – Must be obtained if the medical procedure or treatment involves a material risk of harm to the patient.
- **Malpractice** – The legal term for when a health care professional owes a duty to a patient, breaches that duty, and the patient suffers damages that are proximately caused by the breach of duty.
- **Medical Battery** – The legal claim against a physician if either the patient isn't aware that the physician was going to perform the procedure or the patient hasn't authorized it.
- **Negligence** – A breach of duty based upon the defendant's violation of a statute or regulation.
- **Nonmaleficence** – An obligation to prevent harm or, if risks of harm must be taken, to minimize those risks.

- **Physician-Patient Relationship** – The basis of all legal and ethical obligations between a physician and a patient.
- **Tort** – A civil wrong. It can be intentional or negligent.

PATIENT CONFIDENTIALITY

Protection of patient information is a vital aspect of an EKG Technician's role. Discussion of patient information must be limited to "a need to know basis" and not provided to unauthorized person's not directly involved in the care of the patient. The following describes the Health Information Portability and Accountability ACT (HIPAA) which is a government program developed to protect the patient's privacy.

HEALTH INFORMATION PORTABILITY AND ACCOUNTABILITY ACT (HIPAA)

What Information Is Affected?

Protected Health Information
HIPAA applies to all individually identifiable health information or "protected health information" (PHI) that is transmitted or maintained in electronic or paper records. HIPAA applies to oral communications as well. For example, the rule would cover computer patient profiles, paper prescription orders, telephone conversation with a physician, etc.

Who Is Affected?

Covered Entities
HIPAA applies to health plans, health care clearinghouses, and certain health care providers. Health care providers are covered entities under the regulation if they "transmit any health information in electronic form in connection with a transaction covered by this subchapter." As a health care provider, you have to determine if you conduct any transactions in electronic form. These transactions include: "The transmission of information between two parties to carry out financial or administrative activities related to health care" such as:

1. Health care claims or equivalent encounter information
2. Health care payment and remittance advice
3. Patient Medical Records
4. Patient treatment review or results
5. Patient diagnostic testing results
6. Care Plan reviews
7. Patient demographic/health information
8. Referral certification and authorization
9. Other transactions that the Secretary may prescribe by regulation

If you do not conduct any of the above transactions in electronic form, you are not considered a covered entity under the HIPAA privacy regulation.

WHAT ARE THE NEW REQUIREMENTS?

Interactions with Patients

Notice of Privacy Practices

Covered entities are required to develop and distribute a Notice of Privacy Practices that describes each purpose for which you may use or disclose PHI. The Notice of Privacy Practices must be written in plain language, and it must contain the following information:

- Patient health information rights
- Examples of how the your facility may use and disclose PHI
- Other uses and disclosures of PHI
- Information on how to report a problem
- Effective date

Patient Authorization for Disclosures Not Involving or Outside of Treatment, Payment, and Health Care Operations

A covered health care provider must obtain patient authorization prior to any use or disclosure of protected health information that does not involve treatment, payment, or health care operations. Patient authorization must be in writing, be a separate document from the Notice of Privacy Practices, be written in plain language, and contain the following information:

- Statement that the patient may revoke the authorization in writing to the extent that the information has not already been disclosed;
- Patient's signature and date of signature;
- Description of the information to be used or disclosed;
- Name of the covered entity/provider and the names of any entities authorized to make use or disclosure;
- Name or type of recipient receiving the information;
- Expiration date;
- Notification that once the information is used or disclosed in accordance with the authorization, it may be subject to re-disclosure by the recipient and it may no longer be protected;
- If the authorization is signed by a representative of the patient, the representative must indicate his authority to act for the patient.

Health care providers may <u>not</u> refuse to provide treatment if the patient declines to sign an authorization form. Health care providers must retain authorization forms for a period of 6 years.

PATIENT SAFETY

- Patient Safety: Actions undertaken by individuals and organizations to protect health care recipients from being harmed by the effects of health care services.
- The basic principles for patient safety are the principles for quality of care: to do the right thing for the right patient using the right method and at the right time, and to communicate well with the patient and the rest of the clinical team—record findings, plan actions promptly and clearly, ensure that instructions are understood and carried out, and report concerns to a senior colleague when necessary.
- These principles sound very simple, but most of the serious patient incidents result from a sequence of small errors or failures to act, rather than one large dramatic event. Many errors are the result of human error

- Human errors occur because of:
  - Inattention
  - Memory lapse
  - Failure to communicate
  - Poorly designed equipment
  - Exhaustion
  - Ignorance
  - Noisy working conditions
  - A number of other personal and environmental factors
- What you do?
  - Keep your area free of obstacles and trip hazards
  - Check your equipment for malfunctions or worn wires
  - Assist your patient when necessary
  - Double check your policies and follow them every time
  - Maintain a clean, safe, infection free area

Chapter 7

The EKG
Technician Program
Student Handout #6

ARRHYTHMIAS

Arrhythmias are categorized into groups based on which pacemaker site initiates the rhythm. In a normal rhythm, the electrical impulse originates in the SA node, travels through the internodal tract to cause the atria to contract. The impulse then travels to the AV node, through the AV bundle and into the bundle of HIS. The bundle of HIS then splits into two sections. The left bundle branch travels around the left ventricle and into the purkinje fibers. The right branch travels around the right ventricle and ends in the purkinje fibers. Once the impulse reaches the purkinje fibers, the ventricles then contract forcing the blood out of the heart.

Due to damage in the myocardium, this impulse can originate in other areas of the heart muscle causing the heart to pump ineffectively.

The EKG tracing provides a multitude of clues as to what is happening in the heart. These clues include wave configurations, rates, measurements, and wave relationships. Experts have compiled this data and found that each cardiac arrhythmia has its own set of clues. That is, each specific arrhythmia will repeatedly give off the same set of clues. By looking at the clues available on the strip, you can tell what the rhythm is, but only if you know in advance the kinds of clues that any specific arrhythmia is known to produce. The charts in your study packet give the characteristics common to each arrhythmia.

The following briefly describes common arrhythmias.

Sinus Arrhythmias

- **Normal Sinus Rhythm** – Technically speaking this is not an arrhythmia because it is normal. In normal sinus rhythm, the pacemaker originates in the sinus node and travels through the normal conduction pathways within normal time frames
- **Sinus Bradycardia** – this rhythm follows all of the rules for normal sinus rhythm except for the rate. In this rhythm the rate is lower than 60 bpm
- **Sinus Tachycardia** – The same thing is true for this in that it fits all of the rules for normal sinus rhythm except that the rate is too fast. In this arrhythmia, the rate will be greater than 100 bpm
- **Sinus Arrhythmia** – This rhythm is characterized by a pattern that would normally be considered NSR, except that the rate changes with the patient's respirations. When the patient breathes in, the rate increases and when the patient breathes out, the rate decreases.

Atrial Arrhythmias

- **Wandering pacemaker** – occurs when the pacemaker role switches from beat to beat from the SA node to the atria and back again. The resulting rhythm is made up of interspersed sinus and atrial beats
- **Ectopics** – When a single beat arises from an ectopic focus (a site outside of the SA node) within the conduction system, that beat is called an ectopic beat. When it occurs from the atria it is called an atrial ectopic. An ectopic beat arises when a site somewhere along the conduction system becomes irritable and overrides the SA node for a single beat.
- **Premature Atrial Contraction (PAC)** – A PAC is an ectopic beat that comes early in the cardiac cycle and originates in the atria. Since the PAC comes early in the cardiac cycle, it will usually fall very close to the end of the preceding QRS complex.
- **Atrial Tachycardia** – This arrhythmia is characteristically very regular. It is usually very rapid with a rate of 150–250 bpm. This occurs when a single focus in the atria becomes so irritable that it begins to fire very regularly and thus overrides the SA node for the entire rhythm
- **Atrial Flutter** – When the atria become so irritable that they fire faster than 250 bpm, they are said to be fluttering. It is theorized that an area in the atrium initiates an impulse that is conducted in a repetitive, cyclic pattern, creating a series of atrial waves with a saw-tooth appearance.
- **Atrial Fibrillation** – This rhythm results when the atria become so irritable that they are no longer beating, but merely quivering ineffectively.

Junctional Rhythms

- The AV junction includes the AV node and the Bundle of His.
- When the AV junction assumes pacemaking responsibility the atria and the ventricles will be depolarized at very nearly the same time because the impulse spreads in two directions at one time
- With retrograde conduction to the atria, the P waves will be inverted due to the flow of electrical current towards a negative electrode in Lead I, III and aVF
- The QRS remains upright because this electrical flow is towards a positive electrode
- Inverted P waves can occur before, during or after the QRS.
- When measurable, the PRI will usually measure 0.12 seconds or less
- The AV junction may assume responsibility for pacing the heart if:
  - The SA node fails to discharge
  - An impulse from the SA node is generated but blocked as it exits the SA node (SA block)
  - The rate of discharge of the SA node is slower than that of the AV junction
  - An impulse from the SA node is generated and is conducted through the atria but is not conducted to the ventricles (AV block)

Premature Junctional Contraction

- Arises from an ectopic focus within the AV junction that discharges before the next expected sinus beat
- QRS will usually measure 0.10 or less due to normal conduction thru the ventricles
- Typically an incomplete pause follows so that the SA node can reset itself
- PJC's are distinguished from PAC's by the P wave, PAC typically has an upright P wave before the QRS in leads II, III, aVF
- A P wave may or may not be present with a PJC if present; the P wave will be inverted. It may also be found before, within and behind the QRS. They are less common than a PAC or PVC

Junctional Escape Rhythm

- Junctional escape rhythm originates in the AV junction and appears late as a protective mechanism when the SA node fails to pace or AV conduction fails
- Frequently occur during episodes of sinus arrest or following pauses of nonconducted PAC's
- May be observed in healthy individuals during sinus bradycardia
- Seen in acute MI (Inferior wall)
- Seen in rheumatic heart disease, valvular disease, disease of SA node, hypoxia, increased parasympathetic tone, post CABG, pt's taking dig., quinidine, beta blockers, or calcium channel blockers

Accelerated Junctional Rhythm

- Ectopic rhythm caused by enhanced automaticity of the bundle of His
- Results in ventricular response of 60–100 beats /min
- The ECG criteria is the same as junctional escape except with accelerated junctional rhythm there is an increased ventricular rate

Junctional Tachycardia

- Three or more sequential PJC complexes occurring at a rate of more than 100 beats/min
- Paroxysmal junctional tachycardia describes a tachycardia that starts and ends suddenly and is often precipitated by a premature junctional complex
- When junctional rate is above 100, it is difficult to distinguish from atrial tachycardia and may be called SVT

AV HEART BLOCKS

- If a delay or a block occurs in the AV node, bundle of His, or the purkinje system, the resulting dysrhythmia is called an AV block
- **PRI IS THE KEY TO DIFFERENTIATING THE TYPE OF BLOCK**
- Nothing wrong with the SA node

First Degree AV Heart Block

- Usually all components of the ECG are normal except the PRI
- Caused by a delay at the AV node
- Not a true "block" as all sinus beats are conducted
- PRI greater than .20
- Mild prolongation of the PRI may be a normal variant, occurring especially with physiologic sinus bradycardia during rest or sleep
- 5–10% of pts with AMI have it at some point during the peri-infarct period
- Often asymptomatic, can lead to symptoms
- Monitor closely for pt with acute MI

2nd Degree AV Heart Blocks

2nd Degree type I (Wenckebach, Mobitz Type I)

- Usually occurs at the level of the AV node
- Impulses generated by the SA node take longer and longer to conduct through the AV node, appearing on the ECG as lengthening PR intervals, then resulting in a dropped QRS with a preceding P wave

- Vent. Rhythm is irregular due to the dropped beat
- The pattern repeats itself- must run long strip
- May only prolong one beat then the next will be dropped
- Associated with AV nodal ischemia secondary to occlusion of the RCA
- Usually transient resolving within 48 to 72 hours when associated with an AMI
- May progress to a complete block
- Asymptomatic because the ventricular rate often remains nearly normal and cardiac output is not significantly affected

2nd Degree Block Type II (Mobitz type II or Classical)

- Delay occurs below the AV node, either at the bundle of His or more commonly at the level of the bundle branches. More serious than type I
- Frequently progresses to complete heart block
- SA node is generating impulses in a normal manner, P wave occurs at a regular interval across the strip
- Not every P wave is followed by a QRS
- Impulses generated by the SA node are conducted to the ventricles at the same rate appearing on the ECG as a constant PRI
- PRI is usually within normal limits or slightly prolonged
- Because QRS complexes are dropped ventricular rhythm is irregular

Complete AV Heart Block—Third Degree

- First and second degree blocks are incomplete blocks because the AV junction conducts at least some impulses to the ventricles
- Atria and the ventricles beat independently of each other
- Impulses generated by the SA node are blocked before reaching the ventricles
- Block may occur at the AV node, bundle of His, or the bundle branches
- A secondary pacemaker (either junctional or ventricular) stimulates the ventricles, therefore the QRS may be narrow or wide, depending on the location of the escape pacemaker
- Ventricular rate should be regular
- Complete AV block that occurs with an acute ant. MI is often an indication for insertion of a permanent pacemaker
- When precipitated by a MI it is usually preceded by a 2nd degree classical
- When protected by the junction, it is usually more stable than if the escape comes from the ventricles

VENTRICULAR RHYTHMS

- The ventricle is the heart's least efficient pacemaker and normally generates impulses at a rate of 20–40 beats/min
- Ventricles assume responsibility for pacing when:
  - SA node fails to discharge
  - Impulse from the SA node is generated but blocked as it exits the SA node
  - Rate of discharge of the SA node is slower than that of the ventricles
  - Irritable site in either ventricle produces an early beat or rapid rhythm
- Normally depolarization of the ventricle occurs simultaneously but when an ectopic site in the ventricle assumes responsibility for pacing the heart, the electrical impulse bypasses the normal

intraventricular conduction pathway and stimulation of the ventricles occur asynchronously. As a result, ventricular beats and rhythms are typically characterized by QRS complexes that are abnormally shaped and prolonged.

- Ventricular repolarization is also abnormal resulting in ST and T waves in direction opposite that of the QRS complex

Premature Ventricular Contractions (PVCs)

- Arises from an irritable focus within either ventricle
- Premature
- QRS is greater than .12
- A single beat that may occur in patterns: couplets, run or bursts, bigeminy, trigeminy, quadrigeminy
- Uniform PVC – same appearance from the same site
- Multiform PVC – have different appearance from one another

Ventricular Escape Beat/Rhythm (Idioventricular-IVR)

- Occurs after a pause in which the supraventricular pacemakers failed to initiate impulse
- QRS wide/ bizarre and greater than 0.12 and occur late
- Protective mechanism occur at a rate of 20–40 beats per min
- Ventricular escape rhythm or idioventricular rhythm exists when three or more sequential beats occur at a rate of 20–40.
- Rates lower than 20 are sometimes referred to as **agonal rhythm** or a dying heart
- May occur when the SA node and the AV junction fail to initiate and electrical impulse or when the rate of discharge is less than the inherent rate of the ventricles or if a block occurs above the vent.
- May be precipitated by an MI, dig toxicity, metabolic imbalances
- With loss of atrial kick and slow vent. Pt may experience severe hypotension, weakness, disorientation, lightheadedness, or loss of consciousness because of decreased CO.

Accelerated Idioventricular Rhythm (AIVR)

- Occurs when three or more sequential ventricular escape beats occur at a rate of 40–100 beats/min
- P waves are usually absent unless retrograde conduction occurs
- Vent. Rate usually regular with a QRS greater than 0.12 sec
- T wave frequently in the opposite direction of the QRS complex
- Usually a benign escape rhythm that appears when the sinus rate slows and disappears when the sinus rate speeds up
- Often seen during the first 12 hours of a MI and is common after successful reperfusion therapy
- Seen in both anterior and posterior. Wall MI
- Seen in dig. Toxicity, subarachnoid hemorrhage, and in pt's with rheumatic and hypertensive heart disease
- If pt asymptomatic, no treatment necessary.
- If pt symptomatic because of loss of atrial kick, atropine may be ordered in an attempt to block the vagus nerve and stimulate the SA node to overdrive the ventricular rhythm, or transcutaneous pacing may be attempted.
- Meds to suppress the vent. Rhythm should be avoided because this rhythm is protective and often transient, spontaneously resolving on its own

Ventricular Tachycardia (VT)

- Exists when three or more PVCs occur in immediate succession at a rate greater than 100 beats per min.
- May occur as a short run lasting less than 30 seconds (nonsustained)
- May occur with or without a pulse
- Pt may be stable or unstable
- May originate from an ectopic focus in either ventricle
- QRS is wide and bizarre
- P wave bears no relationship to QRS if seen
- Usually regular may be slightly irregular
- When same shape and amplitude called monomorphic when different polymorphic
- Usually associated with heart disease, particularly myocardial ischemia and rarely occurs in pts without underlying structural heart disease
- Most common cause is CAD
- Other causes: cardiomyopathy, cyclic antidepressant overdose, dig toxicity, valvular heart disease, MVP, trauma, acid base imbalance, electrolyte imbalance and increased production of catecholamines (cocaine abuse)
- S&S may include hemodynamic comp. Related to the tachycardia may include shock, chest pain, hypotension, SOB, pulm. Congestion, CHF, acute MI, and or decreased level of consciousness

Torsades de Pointes

- Polymorphic VT associated with a long QT interval
- French for twisting of the points
- Vent. Rate greater than 200 beats/ min
- Is associated with meds or electrolyte disturbances that prolong the QT interval
- Prolonged QTI indicates a lengthened relative refractory period (vulnerable period) that puts the vent at risk for torsades
- Long QT can be congenital or acquired

Asystole

- Total absence of vent. Electrical activity
- Occurs due to extensive myocardial damage, hypoxia, hypo and hyperkalemia, hypothermia, acidosis, drug overdose, vent. Aneurysm, acute respiratory failure or traumatic cardiac arrest
- Confirmation in 2 leads
- Cause of rhythm and transcutaeous pacing

Myocardial Ischemia and Infarction

One of the prime reasons for performing a 12-lead EKG is to assess for myocardial ischemia (insufficient blood supply to the heart muscle), injury or infarction (heart attack). Every cell and every tissue in the body needs oxygen. The heart is no exception. The heart receives oxygenated blood through a series of arteries called coronary arteries. These arteries are called:

- Right coronary artery (RCA)
- Left main coronary artery (LMCA)
- Left anterior descending artery (LAD)
- Left circumflex
- Posterior descending artery

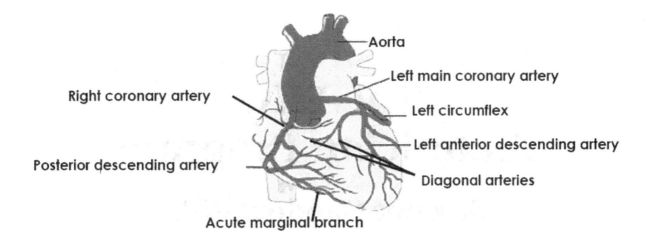

THE PATHOPHYSIOLOGY OF MYOCARDIAL ISCHEMIA, INJURY AND INFARCTION

There are three degrees of hypoxia in tissues: ischemia, injury, and infarction. If injury is present, so is ischemia. If infarction is present, ischemia and injury are also—like a big bruise; purple on the inside, gradually getting lighter on the outer edges.

- Ischemia is the result of inadequate blood or oxygen supply to the myocardium.
- Injury is the second degree of hypoxia
- Infarction is the final degree of hypoxia and means that the cells die from lack of blood supply or oxygen. The area of death becomes electrically silent, causing the electrode on the EKG that faces the area to record an abnormal negative deflection.

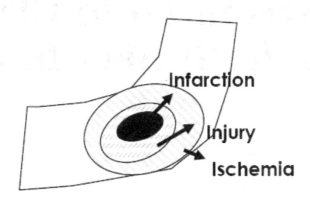

The EKG
Technician Program

Student Handout #6A

Note: See Separate Handout 6A to be Distributed in Class "Arrhythmia Chart"

The EKG Technician Program
Student Handout #7

ECHOCARDIOGRAPHY

Definition

An echocardiogram (or "echo") is a painless test that uses high-frequency sound waves (ultrasound) to get a picture of the heart chambers and valves. The sound waves bounce back from the heart, producing images and sounds that can be used by the physician to detect damage and disease. It is also called a transthoracic echocardiogram. The word "transthoracic" means "across the chest."

Conditions Diagnosed with Echocardiograms

The three most common types of echocardiograms (one-dimensional, two-dimensional and Doppler) are <u>noninvasive</u> and are particularly useful for diagnosing the following conditions:

- **Valvular heart disease.** Types of this disease include a condition in which the valves have narrowed (<u>valvular stenosis</u>: mitral stenosis, aortic stenosis, tricuspid stenosis, or pulmonic stenosis), and a condition in which the valves are leaking (<u>valvular regurgitation</u>: mitral regurgitation, aortic regurgitation, tricuspid regurgitation or pulmonic regurgitation).
- **Rheumatic heart disease.** The effects of rheumatic fever that contribute to major problems with the heart's valves, chambers and vessels.
- **Bacterial endocarditis.** An infection in one or more of the heart valves.
- **Cardiomyopathy.** A disease in which the heart muscle is unusually thick, stiff, dilated or weak.
- **Heart failure.** A condition in which blood flow and circulation are not adequately maintained by one or more valves or chambers of the heart.
- **Pericarditis.** Inflammation of the <u>pericardium</u> (a thin, fluid-filled sac surrounding the heart).
- **Tumors in the heart.**
- **Coronary artery disease.** The obstruction of blood flow to the heart and the body due to hardened arteries (<u>atherosclerosis</u>).
- **Cardiac ischemia.** A condition in which the heart is not getting enough oxygen, usually because blood flow is restricted by hardened arteries (atherosclerosis).
- **Heart attack.** Scarring, or death, of heart muscle due to oxygen deprivation from a closed artery.

- **Shunt.** Abnormal connection between the heart's chambers.
- **Pulmonary hypertension.** <u>High blood pressure</u> (hypertension) in the blood vessels that supply oxygen-poor blood to the <u>lungs</u>.

The physician may also do a stress echocardiogram or "stress echo" to see how the heart functions during physical activity. Usually, a stress echocardiogram involves doing the echocardiogram while the patient is exercising on either a treadmill or a stationary bicycle, at varying speeds and elevations. However, if the patient is unable to perform this physical activity, the physician may choose instead to do a chemical (e.g., dobutamine) stress echocardiogram. This is a test in which the patient is given a medication that causes the heart to beat more strongly, showing the physician what the heart would be doing if it were beating under the more standard stress of exercise.

In addition to diagnosing cardiovascular conditions, there is growing evidence of the usefulness of echocardiograms in assessing the future risk of a coronary event (e.g., heart attack). Researchers have found that in combination with established risk factors, certain echocardiogram findings indicate increased risk. This combined approach may be more effective in identifying people at high risk. Such use of echocardiograms is not yet common, but is likely to gain in popularity as more research is conducted.

During a Noninvasive Echocardiogram

An echocardiogram can be performed in a variety of settings, including hospitals, cardiac labs, testing centers or the physician's office. Most tests take about 30 minutes. Stress echocardiograms (both exercise and chemical) may take up to 1–1/2 hours. Additional time may also be needed for the physician or technician to record information about the patient and to answer all of the patient's questions. Patients are required to remove clothing from the waist up, and are given a hospital gown to wear during the test. The physician or technician will prepare the chest area by applying a conductive gel. People scheduled for a chemical stress echocardiogram will receive an intravenous (I.V.) line via a needle inserted into a vein at the back of the wrist. The I.V. line allows medications to be given to the patient without having to stick the patient with more needles.

A hand-held device called a transducer is then placed on the chest directly over the gel and pictures of the chest are seen immediately on a video monitor. At that time, the lights in the examination room may be dimmed to allow a better view of the various monitors that are recording the results of the echocardiogram.

An electrocardiogram (EKG) may also be performed during this test. The EKG gives information about the electrical activity of the heart and can help detect abnormal heart rhythms (arrhythmias).

A trained sonographer performs the test, and a physician interprets the results. An instrument that transmits high-frequency sound waves called a transducer is placed on the patient's ribs near the breast bone and directed toward the heart. The transducer picks up the echoes of the sound waves and transmits them as electrical impulses. The echocardiography machine converts these impulses into moving pictures of the heart.

Echocardiogram works well for most patients and allows doctors to see the heart beating and to visualize many of the structures of the heart. Occasionally, because the lungs, ribs, or body tissue may prevent the sound waves and echoes from providing a clear picture of heart function, the sonographer may administer a small amount of a dye through an IV to better see the inside of the heart.

How the Test Will Feel to the Patient

The patient will feel a slight pressure on their chest from the transducer. The patient may be asked to breathe in a certain way or to roll over onto their left side.

TYPES OF ECHOCARDIOGRAPHY

There are many different types of echocardiograms, which include the following:

- One-dimensional (M-mode; motion mode). A one-dimensional view of the heart, as if a line were drawn straight through it. This can be black-and-white and/or color.
- Two-dimensional (cross-sectional). A two-dimensional view of the heart, which shows both length and width of heart structures. This can be black-and-white and/or color.
- Three-dimensional echocardiography (3DE). A new technique that may offer superior measurements of the left ventricle, evaluation of areas of the heart muscle vulnerable to damage from heart disease, and assessment of valvular structure and function.

Noninvasive Procedures

Transthoracic Echocardiography (TTE)

This is the most common type of echocardiography exam. It allows the doctors to view the heart from outside the chest without any discomfort to the patient. It does not require the patient to be sedated.

This exam is performed by placing a microphone-shaped device called a transducer on the patient's chest. This transducer sends ultrasound waves over the different areas of the heart, which are reflected back through the transducer and converted into images. One-dimensional images of depth (M-mode) and two-dimensional images of depth and width (2-D) give a picture of the size and structure of the heart, as well as how well it is able to pump, if there are any large clots or tumors within the chambers or if there is any fluid surrounding the heart. Doppler studies (which show the direction and speed of blood flow) can diagnose leaky or tight valves and holes between the different heart chambers and can estimate pressures in the heart and lung circulation. These images are transferred to paper, tape or disc for further interpretation and stored as part of the medical record.

Invasive Procedures

Transesophageal Echocardiography (TEE)

This echocardiography exam uses a very slender, flexible tube that contains the imaging transducer at the tip. This tube is passed through the mouth into the esophagus, where ultrasound pictures are collected from a different angle (posterior view) than are seen with the transthoracic exam (anterior view). The patient is generally lightly sedated to ensure comfort during the procedure. This examination is used to diagnose abnormal heart valves, blood clots, heart infections and aneurysms of the heart and the aorta (the main heart artery), which are sometimes difficult to see with other tests.

Intravascular Ultrasound (IVUS)

This echocardiographic exam is performed in the Cardiac Catheterization Laboratory in conjunction with interventional cardiologists. This procedure uses a catheter that produces ultrasound images of the inside of blood vessels. It is used, along with other imaging modalities, in the catheterization laboratory to look at coronary artery blockages and to see how well different treatments for those blockages are working.

Summary

Each type of echocardiogram provides unique information to the physician regarding the heart structures and function. For example, a one-dimensional echocardiogram is very helpful in determining the size of one of the heart's chambers (atria and ventricles), thickness of the chamber walls, function of the mitral valve and weight of the left ventricle.

The two-dimensional echocardiogram is particularly helpful in seeing the relation of the heart's chambers to each other, the ejection fraction (a measurement of the strength of the left ventricle), and problems with the heart's valves. Doppler ultrasound and its colorized version (the color Doppler) are helpful in detecting a variety of problems, including those of the valves or functional structure below the valves. Doppler can also be an effective tool in screening for pulmonary hypertension in people at risk for developing the condition (e.g., patients with sickle cell anemia).

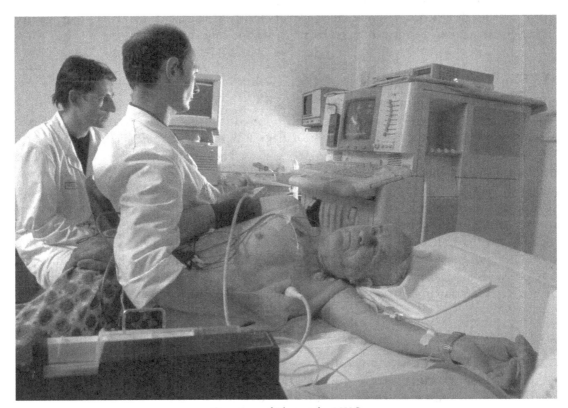

Courtesy of Phototake NYC

The EKG Technician Program

Student Handout #8

STUDY GUIDE

TABLE OF CONTENTS

NOTE * The following information is not exhaustive. It is important that students also study all materials discussed in class in addition to the materials addressed below.

ANATOMY OF THE HEART

- The heart is a hollow muscular organ located in the thoracic cavity between the lungs just behind the sternum. This area of the body is called the mediastinum.
- The heart is a hollow muscular organ about the size of a man's fist.
- The top of the heart is called the base and is broad in shape. It is located just below the 2nd rib on the right side. The bottom of the heart is pointed and called the apex. It lies on the diaphragm.
- The heart functions as a pump to pump blood to all the body's cells. Blood receives oxygen in the lungs when it passes through the alveoli and capillaries in the lungs

Layers of the heart – the heart has three layers that are all fused together and work as a single muscle. These layers are contained in a sac called the pericardium

- *Endocardium* – the innermost layer of the heart. It forms the lining and forms the four valves. It is in this layer that the conduction system is found.
- *Myocardium* – the middle and contractile layer of the heart. It is commonly referred to as the muscle layer of the heart.
- *Epicardium* – the outermost layer of the heart.
- *Pericardium* – a sac in which the heart is contained. It has 2 layers and between these layers is a serous fluid which serves to prevent friction as the heart beats.

The Heart Chambers

- The receiving chambers of the heart are the right atrium and left atrium and the two chambers that push the blood out of the heart called the left and right ventricles. The heart is actually a two-sided pump separated by a septum. The upper chambers consist of the right and left atria and the lower chambers are the right and left ventricles. The chambers pump simultaneously – both atria contract together then the two ventricles.
- Left ventricle – largest chamber of the heart because it pushes the blood out of the heart throughout the body. It also has the largest muscle mass.

Circulation within the Heart

- *Right Atrium* – receives deoxygenated blood returning to the heart from the body via the superior vena cava which carries blood from the upper body and the inferior vena cava which carries blood from the lower body. Deoxygenated blood travels from the right atrium through the tricuspid valve into the right ventricle
- *Right ventricle* – receives deoxygenated blood from the right atrium which it pumps to the lungs for oxygenation through the pulmonary artery to the right and left pulmonary arteries. In the lungs blood travels to Alveoli where the exchange of CO_2 and O_2 are completed. The pulmonary arteries are the only arteries in the body the carry deoxygenated blood.
- *Left atrium* – receives oxygenated blood returning from the lungs via the right and left pulmonary veins. The pulmonary veins are the only veins in the body that carry oxygenated blood. Oxygenated blood then travels from the left atrium through the bicuspid or mitral valve into the left ventricle.
- *Left ventricle* – receives the oxygenated blood from the left atrium and pumps it to the body through the aortic valve into the aorta which is the largest artery of the body.

The Heart Valves – The purpose of the heart valves is to prevent backflow of blood through the heart.

- Atrioventricular valves (AV): so-called because they are located between the atria and ventricles.
  - Tricuspid valve – located between the right atrium and the right ventricle. As the name connotes, it has three cusps.
  - Mitral valve – located between the left atrium and the left ventricle. It has two cusps and it also called the bicuspid valve.
  - The AV valves (mitral and tricuspid valves) are held in place by chordae tendinea.
- Semilunar valves: called semilunar because they have half-moon shaped cusps
  - Pulmonic valve – located between the right ventricle and the pulmonary artery.
  - Aortic valve – located between the left ventricle and aorta
- Murmurs are caused by diseases of the valves or other structural abnormalities.
- Heart failure is most commonly caused by high blood pressure. The top number of the blood pressure called the systolic measures the amount of pressure that is put on the arteries when the left ventricle is contracting. The bottom number of the blood pressure is called the diastolic and measures the amount of pressure put on the heart when the left ventricle is relaxing. A normal BP is 120/80.
- The heart sounds are produced by the closure of the valves:
  S1 – first heart sound is due to the closure of the mitral and tricuspid valves.
  S2 – second heart sound is due to the closure of the aortic and pulmonic valves.

Vessels of the Heart

The arteries supplying the heart are the right and left coronary arising from the first branch of the aorta. These vessels are about 1/8th of an inch in diameter. The veins accompany the arteries, and terminate in the right atrium.

Neural Influences of the Heart

The heart is influenced by the autonomic nervous system (ANS) which is subdivided into the sympathetic and parasympathetic nervous systems.

- Sympathetic nervous system: affects both the atria and the ventricles by increasing heart rate, conduction and irritability.
- Parasympathetic nervous system: affects the atria only by decreasing heart rate, conduction and irritability.

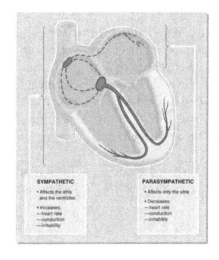

Human Heart

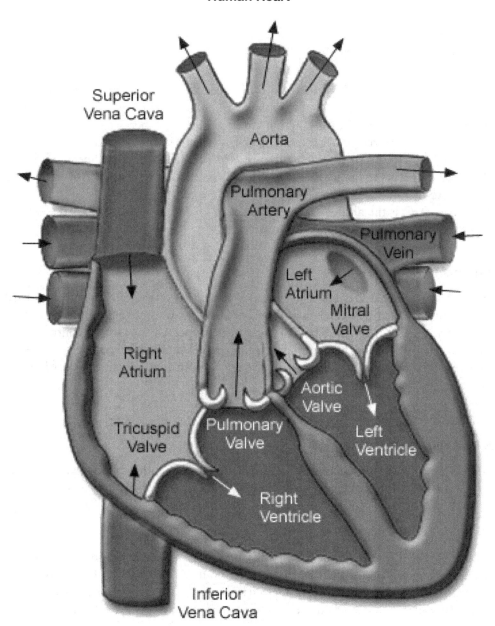

Basic Electrophysiology

Properties of Cardiac Cells

The primary characteristics of the cardiac cells are:

- *Automaticity* – This is the ability of the cardiac pacemaker cells to spontaneously initiate their own electrical impulse without being stimulated from another source. Sites that possess this characteristic are the SA node, AV junction, and the Purkinje fibers.
- *Excitability* – Also referred to as irritability. This characteristic is shared by all cardiac cells and it is the ability to respond to external stimulus: electrical, chemical, and mechanical.
- *Conductivity* – This is the ability of all cardiac cells to receive an electrical stimulus and transmit the stimulus to the other cardiac cells.
- *Contractility* – This is the ability of the cardiac cells to shorten and cause cardiac muscle contraction in response to an electrical stimulus.

Depolarization and Repolarization

Resting cardiac cells are negatively charged inside as compared to the outside. When a cardiac cell is stimulated, sodium ions rush into the cell and potassium leaks out, changing into positive the charge within. This electrical event is called **depolarization** and is expected to result in contraction.

During cell recovery, ions shift back to their original places and the cell recovers the negative charge inside. This is **repolarization,** and proceeds from the epicardium towards the endocardium. It results in myocardial relaxation.

Conduction System of the Heart

SA Node – Found in the upper right atrial wall just below the opening of the superior vena cava. It is the primary pacemaker of the heart and has a normal firing rate of 60–100 beats per minute.

Internodal pathways – Distribute electrical impulse generated by the SA node throughout the right and left atria to the atrioventricular (AV) node.

AV Junction – AV node is located on the lower wall of the right atrium between the atrium and the right ventricle. The AV node receives the impulse from the SA node and when it reaches the AV node, the atria contract. There is a 1/10th of a second delay of electrical activity at this level to allow blood to flow from the atria to the ventricles. Because of this delay, the AV node is known as the "Gatekeeper"

Bundle of His – Found at the top of the interventricular septum, it receives the impulse from the AV node and begins the process that allows the ventricles to contract. It has an ability to initiate electrical impulses with an intrinsic firing rate of 40–60 beats per minute.

Bundle Branches – Runs along each side of the septum along the ventricles. The bundle of His divides into the right and left bundle branches, their function is to conduct the electrical impulses to the Purkinje fibers.

Purkinje fibers – found within the ventricular endocardium, it consists of a network of small conduction fibers that delivers the electrical impulses to the ventricular myocardium. The network has the ability to initiate electrical impulses and act as a pacemaker if higher pacemakers such as the SA or Av nodes fail. The intrinsic firing rate is 20–40 beats per minute.

Conduction System of the Heart

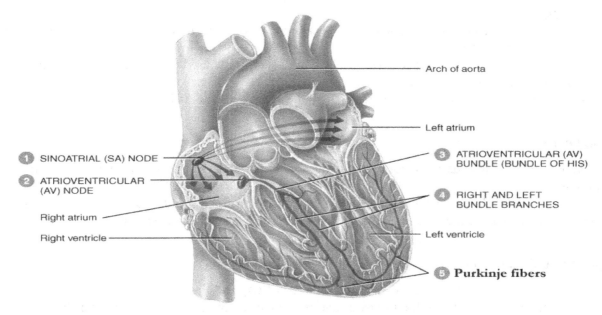

Anterior view of frontal section

Fundamentals of Electrocardiogram

An electrocardiogram is a recording or tracing of an EKG. An electrocardiograph is the machine that records an EKG. An EKG is done with 10 color coded leads. Leads are electrodes that are attached to patients. Electrodes have a substance called electrolyte that helps to pick up the electric current from the skin. The chest leads are called precordial leads. The limb leads are called augmented leads. If a patient has an amputated arm, place the Left and Right arm leads on the Left and Right shoulder area.

Order of Impulse

SA to AV to Bundle of His down the Right and Left Bundle Branches ending in the Purkinje Fibers

The Cardiac Cycle

The cardiac cycle equals one complete heart beat. The parts of the EKG related to the cardiac cycle are:

- P-Q-R-S-T-U segments and waves. If the heart is in normal sinus rhythm, the waves/segments would represent the following
  - P wave represents the contraction of the atria
  - PR interval represents the time it takes for the impulse to go through the atria and AV node
  - QRS complex represents the impulse from the AV node to the Purkinje fibers and contraction of the ventricles
  - Q wave may not be seen and represent the first downward deflection
  - R wave is the first upward deflection after the Q wave
  - S wave is the first downward and upward deflection after the R wave
  - T wave represents the recovery of the heart, the recharging of cells and is typically rounded in shape

- The ST segment is the period between the end of the ventricular contraction and the beginning of recovery
- Q-T interval represents the time from the beginning of ventricular contraction and the end of ventricular recovery
- The R-R interval represents one cardiac cycle and is typically used for measuring the rate if the rhythm is regular
- U wave may not be present but if seen may indicate very low potassium

Limb Leads

Consist of three bipolar leads and three augmented leads. These leads record electrical potentials in the frontal plane.

Electrodes are usually applied just above the wrists or upper arms and ankles although the electrical potential recorded will be the same no matter where electrode is placed in the extremity

Bipolar Standard Leads

Electrodes are applied to the left arm (LA), the right arm (RA) and the left leg (LL). Leads are then applied to their respective electrodes. Electrode and lead are also applied to the right leg which acts as a ground (this lead is usually green in color and has no role in production of the electrocardiogram.

Lead I = the left arm is positive and the right arm is negative.
    (LA – RA) – shows the difference in the heart's voltage between the Rt. Arm and Lt. arm
Lead II = the left leg is positive and the right arm is negative.
    (LL – RA) – shows the difference in the heart's voltage between the Rt. arm and the Lt. leg. This is the most common lead as it checks the electrical activity of the heart from the right atrium through the left ventricle
Lead III = the left leg is positive and the left arm is negative.
    (LL – LA) – shows the differences in the heart's voltage between the Lt. arm and Lt. leg

Augmented Unipolar Lead

They are designated as aVR, aVL, and aVF. Their electricity is produced by small impulses and the EKG machine needs to make them larger (augment) them in order to record them. These leads are unipolar and they require only one electrode from one limb to make a lead. The EKG machine uses a midpoint between the two other limbs as a negative reference point.

Lead aVR = the right arm is positive and the other limbs are negative. – Shows the difference in the heart's voltage between the Rt. arm and mid-point of the Lt. arm and Lt. leg
Lead aVL = the left arm is positive and the other limbs are negative. – Shows the difference in the heart's voltage between the Lt. arm and mid-point of the Rt. Arm and Lt. leg
Lead aVF = the left leg (or foot) is positive and the other limbs are negative. – Shows the difference in the heart's voltage between the Lt. arm and mid-point between the Rt. Arm and Lt. arm

Unipolar Precordial Leads

Six positive electrodes are placed on the chest to create Leads V1 through V6. These leads record the heart's voltage from front to the back of the heart. Recorded area is from the central point within the heart to a point on the chest wall where the electrode is placed. They are as follows:

V1: Fourth intercostal space, right sternal border.
V2: Fourth intercostal space, left sternal border.
V3: Between V2 and V4.
V4: Fifth intercostal space, left midclavicular line
V5: Fifth intercostal space, anterior axillary line
V6: Fifth intercostal space, midaxillary line

Precordial Leads

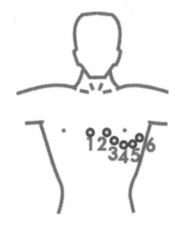

- The usual routine EKG consists of placing 10 electrodes on the patient producing 12 Leads: I, II, III, aVR, aVF, aVL; V1–V6.

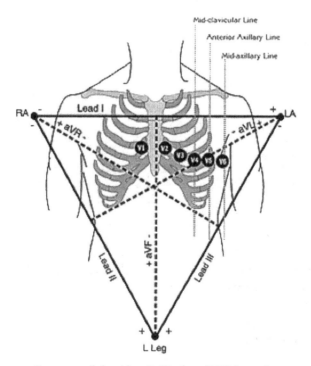

Courtesy of the Alan E. Lindsay EGC Learning
Center in Cyloer Space

The Electrocardiographic Grid

- The EKG paper is a graph paper with horizontal and vertical lines at 1-mm intervals.
- A heavy line appears every 5 mm. The horizontal axis represents time: 1 mm = 0.04 seconds.
- The vertical axis represents amplitude measured in millivolts but expressed in millimeters: 0.1 mV = 1 mm.
- The tracing is marked on the paper by a stylus using heat.
- The running speed is 25 mm/sec. The EKG machine must be properly standardized so that 1 mV will produce a deflection of 10 mm.
- Prior to each EKG a standard check should be performed which should be 10 mm. The standard check represents the voltage of the EKG machine. The standard check should be performed after each EKG as well.

EKG Grid

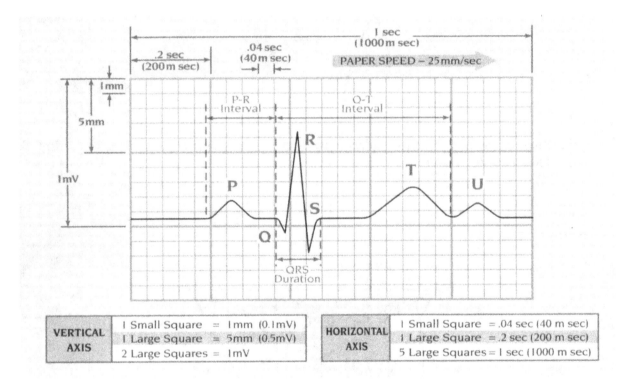

VERTICAL AXIS	1 Small Square = 1mm (0.1mV)		HORIZONTAL AXIS	1 Small Square = .04 sec (40 m sec)
	1 Large Square = 5mm (0.5mV)			1 Large Square = .2 sec (200 m sec)
	2 Large Squares = 1mV			5 Large Squares = 1 sec (1000 m sec)

Waves, Segments and Intervals

- *Waveform*: refers to movement away from the isoelectric line (baseline) either upward (positive) deflection or downward (negative) deflection.
- *Segment*: line between two waveforms.
- *Interval*: waveform plus a segment.
- *Complex*: several waveforms

The Normal Electrocardiogram Complexes

- *Atrial Activation*: P wave: the deflection produced by atrial depolarization. The normal P wave in standard, limb, and precordial leads does not exceed 0.12 s in duration or 2.5 mm in height.
- **Ventricular Activation**: QRS complex: represents ventricular depolarization.
  - *Q (q) wave*: the initial negative deflection produced by ventricular depolarization.
  - *R (r) wave*: the first positive deflection produced by ventricular depolarization.
  - *S (s) wave*: the first negative deflection produced by the ventricular depolarization that follows the first positive deflection, (R) wave.
- **Ventricular Repolarization:**
  - *T wave*: the deflection produced by ventricular repolarization.
  - *U wave*: the deflection seen following the T wave but preceding the next P wave. Prominence is due to hypokalemia (low potassium, blood level).

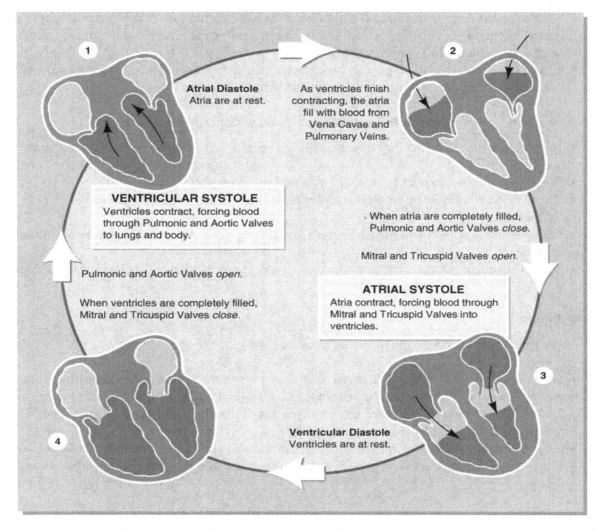

Courtesy of the Walraven. Copyright © 2006 Pearson Education, Inc.

Normal Intervals

RR interval: this is the interval between two R waves. To calculate the heart rate, count the number of R waves in a six second strip and multiply by 10.

Normal Segments and Junctions

- PR segment: line from the end of the P wave to the onset of the QRS complex.
- J (RST) junction: point at which QRS complex ends and ST segment begins.
- ST segment: from J point to the onset of the T wave.

Artifacts

- Somatic tremors – patient's tremors or shaking the wires can produce jittery patterns on the EKG tracing.
- Wandering baseline – sweat or lotion on the patient's skin or tension on the electrode wires can interfere with the signal going to the EKG apparatus causing the baseline of the tracing to move up and down on the EKG paper.
- Broken recording – the stylus goes up and down trying to find the signal. This can be caused by loose electrode or cables or by frayed or broken wires.

Attention to the following will ensure against artifacts and technically poor tracings:

- The patient should be lying on a comfortable bed or table large enough to support the entire body.
- There must be good contact between the skin and the electrode.
- The EKG machine must be properly standardized: 1 mV should produce a deflection of 1 cm (10 mm).
- The patient and the recording machine must be properly grounded to avoid alternating current interference.
- Electronic equipment in contact with the patient can produce artifacts, i.e., IV infusion pumps

Arrhythmias

Cardiac arrhythmias are due to the following mechanisms:

- *Arrhythmias of sinus origin* – where electrical flow follows the usual conduction pathway but is too fast, too slow, or irregular. Normal sinus rate is 60–100 beats per minute. If the rate goes beyond 100 per minute, it is called sinus tachycardia. If the rate goes below 60 per minute, it is referred to as sinus bradycardia.
- *Ectopic rhythms* – electrical impulses originate from somewhere else other than the sinus node.
- *Conduction blocks* – electrical impulses go down the usual pathway but encounter blocks and delays.

Myocardial Ischemia and Infarction

Ischemia

Ischemia occurs when there is a decrease in the amount of blood flow to a section of the heart. This is usually experienced as chest pain and discomfort and is called angina. The lack of sufficient blood supply to the heart muscle can be caused by atherosclerosis which is a buildup of fat deposits in the coronary arteries.

Myocardial Infarction

Infarction refers to the actual death of the myocardial cells. The heart gets its blood from the coronary arteries. The coronary arteries are about 1/8th of an inch in size. If this blood supply stops the heart tissue will die. The steps of a heart attack (also called a MI) are:

- Plaque builds up in the arteries
- A piece of plaque breaks off and the artery wall bleeds creating a clot
- The clot travels through the coronary artery into smaller arteries until it reaches a narrow artery where it is too small to fit through
- The clot plugs the artery and stops the blood flow to the heart muscle
- This describes a heart attack or MI. An EKG is used to diagnose a heart attack.

SINUS ARRHYTHMIAS

Normal Sinus Rhythm

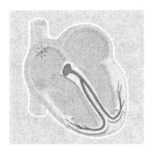

- Regularity: Regular
- Rate: 60–100 beats per minute
- P Wave: Normal and upright; one P wave in front of every QRS complex
- PRI: .12–.20 seconds and constant
- QRS: Less than .12 seconds

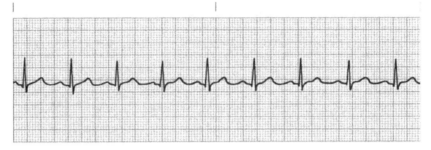

Sinus Bradycardia

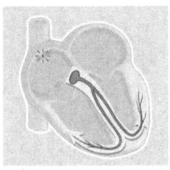

- Regularity: Regular
- Rate: Less than 60 beats per minute
- P Wave: Normal and upright; one P wave in front of every QRS complex
- PRI: .12–.20 seconds and constant
- QRS: Less than .12 seconds

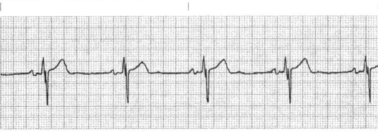

Sinus Tachycardia

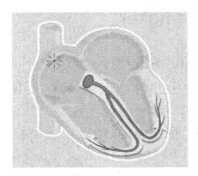

- Regularity: Regular
- Rate: Greater than 100 beats per minute (usually 100–160 beats per minute)
- P Wave: Normal and upright; one P wave in front of every QRS complex
- PRI: .12–.20 seconds and constant
- QRS: Less than .12 seconds

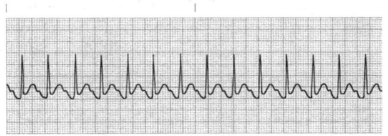

Sinus Arrhythmia

Slide #26

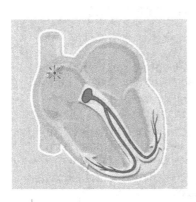

- Regularity: Irregular
- Rate: 60–100 beats per minute (usually)
- P Wave: Normal and upright; one P wave in front of every QRS complex
- PRI: .12–.20 seconds and constant
- QRS: Less than .12 seconds

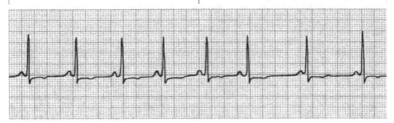

ATRIAL ARRHYTHMIAS

Wandering Pacemaker

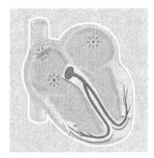

- Regularity: Slightly irregular
- Rate: Usually normal, 60–100 beats/minute
- P Wave: Morphology changes from beat to beat
- PRI: Less than .20 seconds; may vary
- QRS: Less than .12 seconds

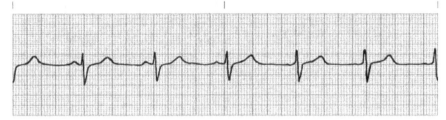

Premature Atrial Contraction

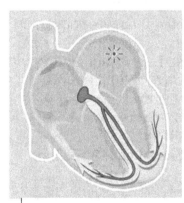

- Regularity: Depends on underlying rhythm; usually regular except for PAC
- Rate: Usually normal; depends on underlying rhythm
- P Wave: P wave of early beat differs from sinus P Waves; can be flattened or notched; may be lost in preceding T wave
- PRI: .12–.20 seconds; can be greater than .20 seconds
- QRS: Less than .12 seconds

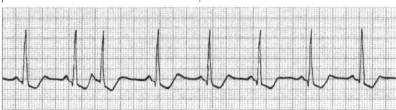

Atrial Tachycardia

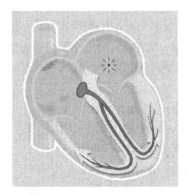

- Regularity: Regular
- Rate: 150–250 beats per minute
- P Wave: Atrial P wave; differs from sinus P wave; can be lost in preceding T wave
- PRI: .12–.20 seconds
- QRS: Less than .12 seconds

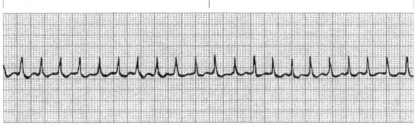

Atrial Flutter

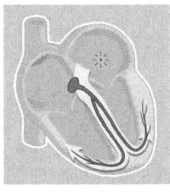

- Regularity: Atrial Rhythm regular; ventricular rhythm usually regular but can be irregular if there is variable block
- Rate: Atrial rate 250–350 beats per minute; ventricular rate varies
- P Wave: Characteristic sawtooth pattern
PRI: Unable to determine
- QRS: Less than .12 seconds

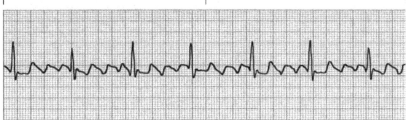

Atrial Fibrillation

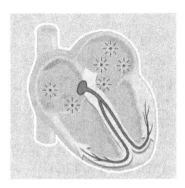

•Regularity: Grossly irregular

•Rate: Atrial greater than 350 beats per minute; ventricular rate varies greatly

•P Wave: No discernible P waves; atrial activity is referred to as fibrillatory waves (f waves)

•PRI: Unable to measure

•QRS: Less than .12 seconds

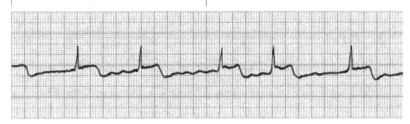

JUNCTIONAL ARRYTHMIAS

Premature Junctional Contraction

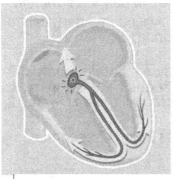

- •Regularity: Depends on rhythm of underlying arrhythmia
- •Rate: Depends on rate of underlying arrhythmia
- •P Wave: Inverted; can fall before, during, or after QRS complex
- •PRI: Can only be measured if P wave precedes QRS complex; if measurable, will be less than .12 seconds
- •QRS: Less than .12 seconds

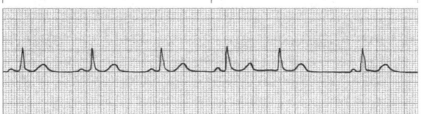

Junctional Escape Rhythm

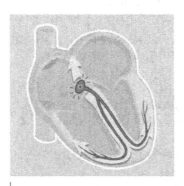

- •Regularity: Regular
- •Rate: 40–60 beats per minute
- •P Wave: Will be inverted; can fall before, during, or after QRS complex
- •PRI: Can be measured only if P wave precedes QRS complex; if measurable, will be less than .12 seconds
- •QRS: Less than .12 seconds

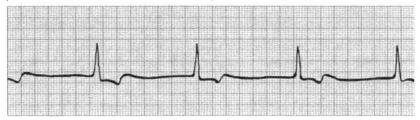

Accelerated Junctional Rhythm

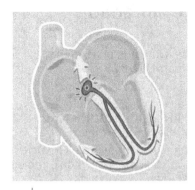

- Regularity: Regular
- Rate: 60–100 beats per minute
- P Wave: Will be inverted; can fall before, during, or after QRS complex
- PRI: Can be measured only if P wave precedes QRS complex; if measurable, will be less than .12 seconds
- QRI: Less than .12 seconds

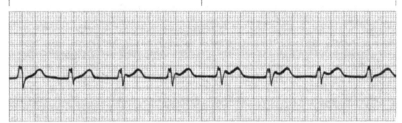

Junctional Tachycardia

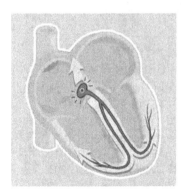

- Regularity: Regular
- Rate: 100–180 beats per minute
- P Wave: Will be inverted; can fall before, during, or after QRS complex
- PRI: Can be measured only if P wave precedes QRS complex; if measurable, will be less than .12 seconds
- QRS: Less than .12 seconds

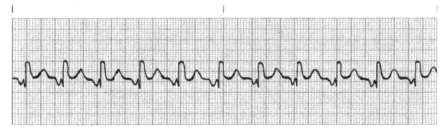

HEART BLOCKS

First Degree Heart Block

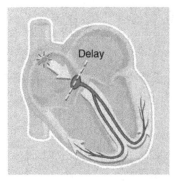

- Regularity: Depends on underlying rhythm
- Rate: Depends on underlying rhythm
- P Wave: Upright and uniform; each P wave followed by QRS complex
- PRI: Greater than .20 seconds; constant across strip
- QRS: Less than .12 seconds

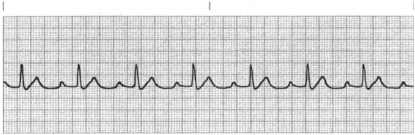

Type II Second Degree Heart Block

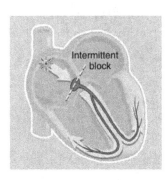

- Regularity: If conduction ratio is consistent, R-R interval will be constant, and rhythm will be regular. If conduction ratio varies, R-R will be irregular.
- Rate: Atrial rate is usually normal. Since many atrial impulses are blocked, ventricular rate is usually bradycardic (often one-half, one-third, or one-fourth the atrial rate).
- P Wave: Upright and uniform; always outnumber QRS complexes.
- PRI: Constant on conducted beats, but possibly prolonged.
- QRS: Less than .12 seconds.

Conduction Ratios in Type II Second Degree Heart Block

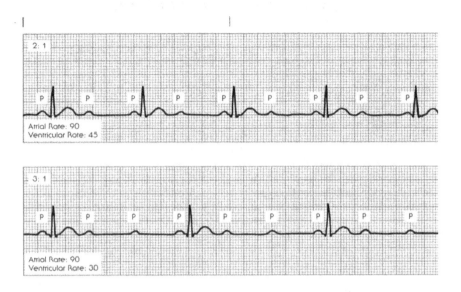

Conduction Ratios in Type II Second Degree Heart Block

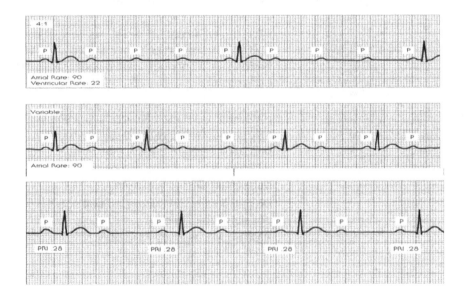

Type I Second Degree Heart Block
(Wenckebach)

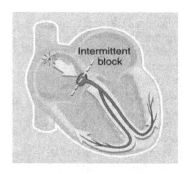

Slide #46

•Regularity: Irregular; R-R interval changes as PR interval gets longer; characteristic grouped beating

•Rate: Usually slightly slower than normal

•P Wave: Upright and uniform; some P waves not followed by QRS complexes

•PRI: Progressively lengthens until one P wave is not conducted

•QRS: Less than .12 seconds

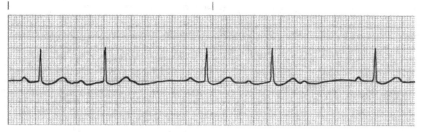

Complete Heart Block

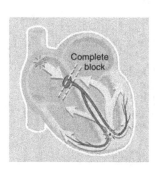

•Regularity: Regular

•Rate: 40–60 beats per minute if focus is functional

         20–40 beats per minute if focus is ventricular

•P Wave: Upright and uniform; more P waves than QRS complexes

•PRI: No relationship between P waves and QRS complexes; P waves occasionally superimposed on QRS complexes

•QRS: Less than .12 seconds if focus is functional; .12 seconds or more if focus is ventricular

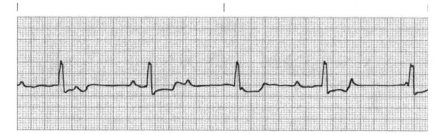

VENTRICULAR ARRYTHMIAS

Premature Ventricular Contractions

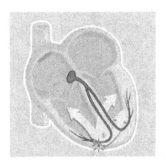

Regularity: Ectopics will disrupt regularity of underlying rhythm

Rate: Depends on underlying rhythm and number of ectopics

P Wave: Not preceded by a P wave; dissociated P waves may be seen near PVC

PRI: Since the ectopic comes from a lower focus, there will be no PRI

QRS: Wide and bizarre; .12 seconds or greater; T wave is usually in opposite direction from R wave

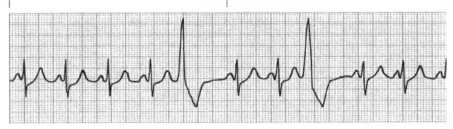

Ventricular Tachycardia

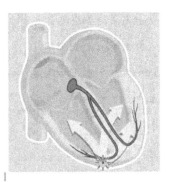

•Regularity: Usually regular; can be slightly irregular

•Rate: Usually 150–250 beats/min; less than 150 is called slow VT; over 250 is called Ventricular Flutter

•P Wave: Not preceded by P waves; dissociated P waves may be seen

•PRI: None

•QRS: Wide and bizarre; .12 sec. or greater

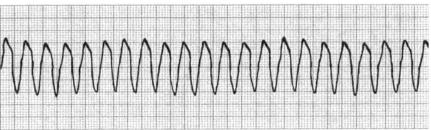

Ventricular Fibrillation

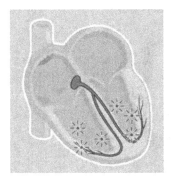

- •Regularity:
- •Rate:
- •P Wave:
- •PRI:
- •QRS:

} Totally chaotic with no discernible waves or complexes

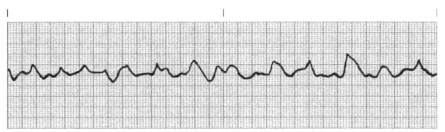

Idioventricular Rhythm

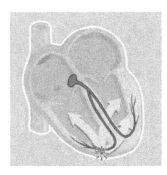

- •Regularity: Usually regular (it can be unreliable since it is such a low site)
- •Rate: 20–40 beats per minute; can drop below 20 beats per minute
- •P Wave: None
- •PRI: None
- •QRS: Wide and bizarre; .12 seconds or greater

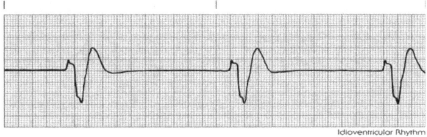

Idioventricular Rhythm

Asystole

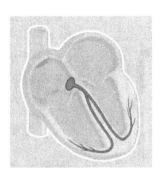

- •Regularity:
- •Rate:
- •P Wave:
- •PRI:
- •QRS:

} Straight line indicates absence of electrical activity

PACEMAKER SPIKES AND CAPTURE

 # Single Chamber Pacemaker

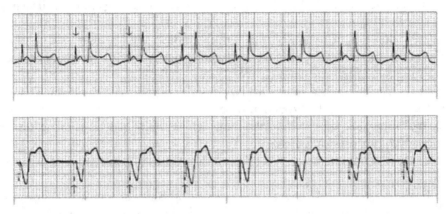

 # Dual Chamber Pacemakers

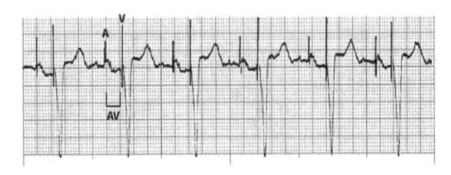

Respiratory System: Oxygen Delivery System

The primary function of the respiratory system is to supply the blood with oxygen in order for the blood to deliver oxygen to all parts of the body. The respiratory system does this through breathing. When we breathe, we inhale oxygen and exhale carbon dioxide. This exchange of gases is the respiratory system's means of getting oxygen to the blood.

Respiration is achieved through the mouth, nose, trachea, and lungs in the following way:

- Oxygen enters the respiratory system through the mouth and the nose.
- The oxygen then passes through the larynx (where speech sounds are produced) and the trachea which is a tube that enters the chest cavity.
- In the chest cavity, the trachea splits into two smaller tubes called the bronchi. Each bronchus then divides again forming the bronchial tubes.
- The bronchial tubes lead directly into the lungs where they divide into many smaller tubes which connect to tiny sacs called alveoli.
- The inhaled oxygen passes into the alveoli and then diffuses through the capillaries into the arterial blood.
- Meanwhile, the waste-rich blood from the veins releases its carbon dioxide into the alveoli.
- The carbon dioxide follows the same path out of the lungs when you exhale.

Anatomy of the Respiratory System

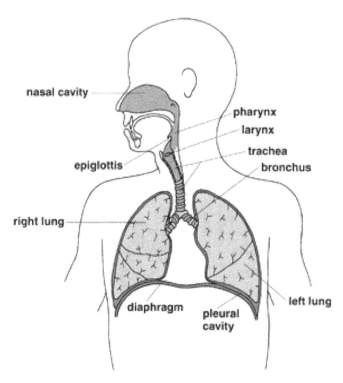

Courtesy of the University of Maryland Medical Center

Primary Function

The primary function of the respiratory system is to obtain oxygen for use by body's cells and eliminate carbon dioxide that cells produce. The following describes the pathway of air through the Respiratory System:

Nasal cavities (or oral cavity) ⟶ Pharynx ⟶ Trachea ⟶ Bronchi (right & left) ⟶ Bronchioles ⟶ Alveoli (site of gas exchange)

The exchange of gases (O_2 & CO_2) between the alveoli & the blood occurs by simple diffusion. Diffusion is the movement of particles from an area of high concentration to an area of low concentration in a given volume of fluid (either liquid or gas). To facilitate diffusion in our lungs, the concentration (or pressure) of O_2 in the alveoli must be kept at a higher level than in the blood and the concentration (or pressure) of CO_2 in the alveoli must be kept at a lower lever than in the blood. We do this, of course, by breathing – continuously bringing fresh air (with lots of O_2 & little CO_2) into the lungs & the alveoli.

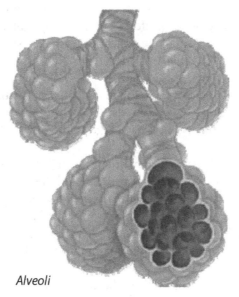

Alveoli

Courtesy of Union County College
Department of Biology

Pulmonary Ventilation

Pulmonary ventilation is commonly referred to as breathing. It is the process of air flowing into the lungs during inspiration (inhalation) and out of the lungs during expiration (exhalation). Air flows because of pressure differences between the atmosphere and the gases inside the lungs. The 3 main phases of respiration are:

- Pulmonary ventilation – inhalation and exhalation
- Diffusion – actual exchange of oxygen and carbon dioxide gases
- Transportation – Oxygen and other nutrients are transported to the cells via the blood and once diffusion takes place, carbon dioxide is transported back to the lungs to drop off the carbon dioxide and pick up oxygen

Average respiratory rate reported in a healthy adult at rest is usually given as 12 breaths per minute with a normal respiration range of 12–20 per minute.

Respiratory Terms

- **Inspiration** – Inspiration (inhalation) is the process of taking air into the lungs. It is the active phase of ventilation because it is the result of muscle contraction. During inspiration, the diaphragm contracts and the thoracic cavity increases in volume. Inspiration draws air into the lungs.
- **Expiration** – Expiration (exhalation) is the process of letting air out of the lungs during the breathing cycle. Expiration pushes air out of the lungs.
- **Ventilation** – The process of breathing.
- **Diffusion** – Diffusion is the movement of particles from an area of high concentration to an area of low concentration in a given volume of fluid (either liquid or gas)
- **Transportation** – the movement of O_2 and CO_2 through the blood and through inspiration and expiration.
- **Respiratory Rate:** The number of breaths the patient takes in one minute. These are counted by the nurse over a period of one minute. It is best done if the patient is not aware that his respiratory rate is being counted. The average adult respiratory rate is 12.
- **Tidal volume:** The amount of air which enters and leaves the lungs during one regular breath.
- **Nasal** – The nose (nasal cavity) is the preferred entrance for outside air into the respiratory system. The hairs that line the wall are part of the air-cleaning system.
- **Pharynx** – The throat (pharynx) collects incoming air from the nose and mouth and passes it downward to the windpipe (trachea).
- **Larynx** – The voice box (larynx) contains the vocal chords. It is the place where moving air being breathed in and out creates voice sounds.
- **Trachea** – The WINDPIPE (trachea) is the passage leading from the throat (pharynx) to the lungs
- **Bronchi** – The windpipe divides into the two main bronchial tubes, one for each lung, which subdivide into each lobe of the lungs. These, in turn, subdivide further.
- **Bronchioles** – The smallest subdivisions of the bronchial tubes are called bronchioles.
- **Alveoli** – very small air sacs that are the destination of air breathed in. Imbedded in the walls of the alveoli are capillaries. Blood passes through the capillaries. While in the capillaries the blood gives off carbon dioxide through the capillary wall into the alveoli and takes up oxygen from the air in the alveoli.
- **Lungs** – The right lung is divided into three lobes, or sections. Each lobe is like a balloon filled with sponge-like tissue. The left lung is divided into two LOBES.

GLOSSARY OF EKG TERMS

Agonal

This is a slow, irregular rhythm with wide ventricular complexes of varying morphology, which is often seen during the later stages of unsuccessful resuscitation attempts as the heart dies.

Angina pectoris

A suffocating pain (angina) of the chest (pectoris). Angina is a result of the oxygen demands of the heart not being met. This can be caused by increased oxygen demand or by decreased oxygen supply.

Aortic arch

The part of the aorta that connects the ascending (just as it leaves the heart) with the descending aorta.

Aortic valve

Valve between the left ventricle and aorta

Apex

Pointed tip of the heart

Arrhythmia

An abnormal heart rhythm, referring to a disruption of the regular rhythmic pattern of the contraction of the heart's chambers, causing the heart to beat too fast, too slow or irregularly

Arteriole

Microscopic blood vessels that connect the smallest arteries with the capillary beds. The arterioles together with the smaller arteries make up the resistance vessels.

Arteriosclerosis

A hardening of medium and large arteries. The most common form of arteriosclerosis is atherosclerosis

Artery

Carries oxygenated blood to the body

Artifact

Waves or lines seen on the EKG that are a result of outside disturbance not from the heart's electrical activity

Asystole

Absence (a) of contraction (systole). Asystole is when the heart has stopped beating. This is different than fibrillation where the heart is still contracting, but not in a coordinated fashion.

Atrial arrhythmia

An abnormal rhythm that develops in the upper chambers (atria) of the heart

Atrial fibrillation (A fib)

An arrhythmia that occurs when the atria contract in a very rapid and irregular fashion

Atrioventricular (AV) node

Specialized conduction tissue found in the right atrium. In a healthy heart the AV node is the only electrical connection between the atria and ventricles. By having a relatively slow conduction rate, the AV node allows the atria to empty more blood into the ventricles before they contract.

Atrium, atria (pl)

The upper chambers of the heart. Blood returning to the heart is stored in the atria before being ejected into the ventricles.

Augmented leads

Unipolar leads that measure electrical flow on the frontal plane from the center of the heart to each of the three limb leads: Leads aVR, aVL, and aVF.

AV Bundle

Also known as the Bundle of HIS, the atrioventricular bundle, is a collection of heart muscle cells specialized for electrical conduction that transmits the electrical impulses from the AV node to the purkinje fibers

AV Junction

The combination of the AV node and the Bundle of His

AV Node

Atrioventricular node (intrinsic rate of 40–60 bpm)

Base

Top of the heart, lies level with the second rib on the right side

Baseline

The isoelectric line on the EKG paper that indicates lack of electrical activity

Bicuspid Valve

The mitral valve, has two cusps or points

Blood Pressure

A measure of pressure on the vessels when the heart is beating (systole) and between beats (diastole).

Bradycardia

Slow (Brady) heart (cardiac). Bradycardia is an abnormally slow heart rate (less than 50 bpm for an adult).

Bundle branches

Bundle of fibers that was divided into 2 branches on either side of the septum along the ventricles; part of the conduction system

Bundle of His

The bundle of fibers that arise from the AV node and lie on the top of the septum; part of the conduction system

Cardiac arrest

The cessation of cardiac function

Cardiac cycle

The interval from the beginning of one heartbeat to the beginning of the next; on the EKG it encompasses the PQRST complex

Cardiac muscle
Myocardium; specialized to conduct an impulse so that it contracts

Cardiac output
The amount of blood per a minute that the heart pumps.

Chordae tendinea
Specialized fibers that connect valve leaflets to papillary muscles to prevent back-flow during contraction

Congestive heart failure (CHF)
A condition when the heart, for whatever reason, cannot meet the demands of the body. The body compensates in three major ways.

Contractility
Contractility refers to how strongly the heart contracts.

Coronary artery
Arising from the first branch of the Aorta and feeds the myocardium

Coronary insufficiency
The right and left coronary arteries supply blood to the heart. Flow is considered insufficient if it cannot meet the needs of the heart. See ischemia.

Depolarization
The electrical process of discharging polarized cells, usually resulting in muscle contraction

Diastole
The period of the cardiac cycle when the ventricles are relaxed. It begins approximately with the opening of the AV valves and ends with their closing. It is during diastole that the ventricles fill with blood.

Ectopic
An adjective referring to an event or tissue occurring at a place other than its normal location. Ectopic heart beats are generated from an impulse originating some other place than the SA node.

Edema
The accumulation of extra fluid in tissues. The tissue looks puffy and if pressed with a finger will hold the indentation after the finger is removed. In CHF when the body starts to retain water to raise the blood pressure, edema can often result. Pulmonary edema (excessive fluid in the lung tissue) can also result.

Electrocardiogram (ECG, EKG)
The report from a test that records the electrical activity of the heart

Electrocardiograph
A test that records the electrical activity of the heart

Electrode
Metal wire attached to the patient's body for the purpose of conveying electrical impulses to a machine for recoding or displaying

Electrolyte gel

Multi-purpose, highly-conductive, water soluble gel that supports the conduction of electrical impulse

Endocardium

The outer layer of the heart

Fibrillation

A nonsynchronous contraction of muscle tissue, with individual cells firing at their own rate. Fibrillation can be isolated to the atria or the ventricles. Ventricle fibrillation is not compatible with life. A heart in fibrillation has been described as looking and feeling like a "bag of worms."

Flutter

An extremely fast heart beat (200–350 bpm) usually occurring only in the atria. Flutter is different than fibrillation in that flutter is a coordinated beat.

Hemostasis

Blood (hemo) stopping of flow (stasis). The termination of bleeding due to clotting and vasoconstriction.

His bundle (bundle of His)

The bundle of His or AV bundle is the part of the Purkinje system that connects directly to the AV node. It later breaks into two separate tracks (right and left bundle branches).

Infarction

The death of tissue due to a lack of blood flow. A myocardial infarction is death of part of the heart muscle caused by an obstruction of a coronary artery.

Inotropic effect/state

Ino- is a prefix that refers to muscle. Inotropic effects are ones that change the strength of contraction of the heart muscle.

Intercostal spaces

The space between two ribs

Intervals

The distance between two points on an EKG

Ischemia

Reduced (isch) blood (emia). A condition of inadequate blood flow to a tissue. Ischemia to the heart can cause angina, and if present long enough, infarction.

Leads

An electrocardiographic view of the heart, gained by recording the electrical activity between two or more electrodes

Mediastinum

The space between the lungs in the chest cavity; holds the heart and other respiratory units

Midaxillary

An imaginary line that passes vertically down the body from the apex of the axilla (armpit).

Midclavicular
An imaginary line that passes vertically down the body from the middle of the clavicle

Mitral valve
a.k.a. Bicuspid valve; on the left side between the atrium and ventricle

Myocardial infarction
Death to an area of the myocardium due to the lack of blood to that area

Myocardium
Heart muscle; middle layer of the heart; specialized cardiac muscles all fused together so that when one part reacts, it all reacts (contracts)

Murmur
An abnormal heart sound most often caused by defective heart valves.

PQRST
The P wave represents atrial depolarization and the QRS represents ventricular depolarization. The T wave reflects the phase of rapid repolarization of the ventricles.

Pacemaker node
a.k.a. SA or Sinoatrial node; impulse is generated here to stimulate the heart to beat

Paroxysmal
Referring to an attack or condition of sudden onset. Paroxysmal tachycardia is a sudden (two to five seconds) increase in heart rate.

Pericardium
Fibrous fluid filled sac that encloses the heart and its blood vessels

Polarization
Refers to a steady state where the electrical charges are balanced and no electrical current flows

Precordial leads
Leads that measure electrical flow on the horizontal plane, from the center of the heart to locations around the anterior and lateral chest walls. The V leads: V1, V2, V3, V4, V5, and V6

Pulmonary artery
Only artery that carries low oxygen blood; leaves right ventricle and goes to the heart

Pulmonary circulation
Circulation that goes to the heart's right atrium to the lungs where it is oxygenated and releases built up carbon dioxide

Pulmonary vein
Only vein that carries high oxygen blood; comes from the lungs and returns blood back to the left atrium for eventual circulation to body organs and cell

Pulmonic valve
The valve that controls the passage of blood from the right ventricle to the pulmonary artery

Purkinje system

The Purkinje fibers are specialized conducting cells found in the ventricular septum of the heart. They transmit the impulse from the <u>AV node</u> to the myocardium. They are organized in such a way as to mediate a smooth contraction that wrings the blood from the apex out toward the base of the heart.

R-R Complex

One complete cardiac cycle

Repolarization

The process of recharging depolarized cells back to their "ready" (polarized) state

Resting phase

Cardiac cells at rest are considered polarized which means no electrical activity takes place

Rheumatic fever

Rheumatic fever is an inflammatory disease that can develop as a rare complication of untreated or undertreated strep throat infection which can result in cardiac valve damage

Sinoatrial (SA) node

Specialized myocardial tissue found in the upper wall of the right atrium. The SA node is the pace maker of the heart. Although other tissues in the heart have intrinsic pacemaker abilities, in a healthy heart the SA node fires at the fastest rate, thereby driving the other tissues.

Segments

The distances between the deflections on an ECG are called segments

Septum

A dividing wall between the right and left sides of the heart.

Sinus rhythm

In the normal heart, heart rate is under the control of the SA node and is said to be in sinus rhythm. Conduction blocks or an ectopic source of impulses can remove the heart from normal sinus rhythm.

Striated

Muscle tissue that is marked by transverse dark and light bands, is made up of elongated usually multinucleated fibers

Superior vena cava

Vein that carries deoxygenated blood from the upper body back to the right atrium

Sympathetic tone

"Fight or flight" response. The sympathetic system prepares the body for action.

- increased heart rate.
- increased contractility.
- increased blood pressure.
- blood flow increased to skeletal muscle.
- blood flow decreased to viscera.
- release of catecholamines by adrenal gland.
- retention of sodium and water (secretion of <u>rennin</u> from the kidney)
- relaxation of bronchiolar smooth muscle.

Syncope

Temporary loss of consciousness due to reduced blood flow to the brain. A common symptom of cardiac arrhythmias.

Systemic circulation

The portion of the cardiovascular system which carries oxygenated blood away from the heart, to the body, and returns deoxygenated blood back to the heart.

Systole

The part of the cardiac cycle when the ventricles are contracting. Systole begins with the closing of the AV valves and ends with their opening.

Tachycardia

Fast (Tachy) heart (cardiac). An abnormally fast heart rate.

Tricuspid valve

A valve that is on the right side of the heart, between the right atrium and the right ventricle.

Vagal tone

Vagal tone is virtually synonymous with parasympathetic tone in regards to the heart. Stimulation of the vagus causes a decreased heart rate, which in turn causes a drop in blood pressure.

Vasoconstriction

The effects of vasoconstriction (or the constriction of a vessel) are best understood if the following relationship is remembered. Resistance through a vessel is inversely proportional to the fourth power of the radius. Simply put, a small decrease in the radius of a vessel can cause a marked decrease in flow or increase in pressure or both.

Vasodilatation

Also known as vasodilatation. It is caused by relaxing the smooth muscle around a vessel, allowing it to increase in diameter. See vasoconstriction.

Ventricle

The two lower chambers of the heart. These two chambers are responsible for sending blood out into the circulation. The left ventricle pumps blood into the systemic circulation and the right ventricle pumps blood into the pulmonary circulation.

Wolff-Parkinson-White syndrome

A conduction disorder of the heart where electrical pathways other than the AV nodal system connect the atria with the ventricles. This type of disorder can lead to reentrant arrhythmias.

PART C
EKG Technician Program

STUDENT GRADUATE ASSISTANCE PACKET

TABLE OF CONTENTS

Note: This packet can be used by students interested in finding employment in health care as well as other related fields. The information in this packet includes helpful hints, best practices, interview techniques and other information to assist students in their search for life long employment.

The EKG Technician Program

INTRODUCTION

Your hands are damp as you wring them uncontrollably. Your mouth is dry, and you wonder if the right words will ever escape you lips. Your stomach is doing loop-de-loops as you make yet another run for the bathroom. And this is only the day before the interview!

Does this sound like you? You're not alone. It is very common, and normal, to be nervous before an interview. Feeling anxious will raise your energy level, and that's a good thing, just be sure you don't get too nervous. The best way to avoid common job search and interview mistakes is to prepare.

This Student Graduate Assistance Packet and any attachments are the confidential property of Condensed Curriculum International Inc.

C-3

The EKG
Technician Program

THE RESUME

Your resume is a tool with one specific purpose: to win an interview. A resume is an advertisement, nothing more, nothing less.

A great resume doesn't just tell them what you have done but makes the same assertion that all good ads do: If you buy this product (Me), you will get these specific, direct benefits. It presents you in the best light. It convinces the employer that you have what it takes to be successful in this new position or career.

It is so pleasing to the eye that the reader is enticed to pick it up and read it. It "whets the appetite," stimulates interest in meeting you and learning more about you. It inspires the prospective employer to pick up the phone and ask you to come in for an interview.

Your cover letter should make the reader want to learn more about you and provide a preview to your resume. It should not provide the same details as your resume but act as an introduction to your resume.

When creating your resume, use the following guidelines:

- **The resume is visually enticing,** a work of art. Simple clean structure. Very easy to read . . . Uncrowded.
- **There is uniformity and consistency in the use of italics, capital letters, bullets, boldface, and underlining** For example, if a period is at the end of one job's dates, a period should be at the end of all jobs' dates.
- **There are absolutely no errors.** No typographical errors. No spelling errors. No grammar, syntax, or punctuation errors. No errors of fact.
- **All the basic, expected information is included.** A resume must have the following key information: your name, address, phone number, and your email address at the top of the first page, a listing of jobs held, in reverse chronological order, educational degrees including the highest degree received, in reverse chronological order. Additional, targeted information will of course accompany this.

- **Jobs listed** include a title, the name of the firm, the city and state of the firm, and the years.
- **It is targeted.** A resume should be targeted to your goal, to the ideal next step in your career.
- **Strengths are highlighted/weaknesses de-emphasized.** Focus on whatever is strongest and most impressive.
- **Use power words.** For every skill, accomplishment, or job described, use the most active impressive verb you can think of (which is also accurate).
- **Show you are results-oriented.** Wherever possible, prove that you have the desired qualifications through a clear strong statement of accomplishments . . . For example: "Initiated and directed complete automation of the Personnel Department, resulting in time-cost savings of over 25%."
- **Writing is concise and to the point.** Keep sentences as short and direct as possible.
- **Make it look great.** Use a laser printer or an ink jet printer that produces high-quality results. Use a standard conservative typeface (font) in 11 or 12 point. Don't make them squint to read it. Use off-white, ivory or bright white 8 1/2 × 11-inch paper, in the highest quality affordable.
- **Shorter is usually better.** Everyone freely gives advice on resume length. Most of these self-declared experts say a resume should always be one page.
- **Break it up.** A good rule is to have no more than six lines of writing in any one writing "block" or paragraph (summary, skill section, accomplishment statement, job description, etc.). If any more than this is necessary, start a new section or a new paragraph.
- **Experience before education . . . usually.** Experience sections should come first, before education, in most every case.
- **Telephone number that will be answered.** Be sure the phone number on the resume will, without exception, be answered by a person or an answering machine Monday through Friday 8–5 p.m.

EMPLOYMENT HISTORY GAPS

What's wrong with a few gaps in my work history?" you might ask. "Isn't everyone entitled to a little time off?" Many responsible professionals have taken breaks in their careers to travel, take care of ill parents, recover from illness, and a myriad of other legitimate projects. But for some reason, employers don't like to see gaps in your work history.

If you have a period of unemployment in your history, here are some ways of dealing with it:

1. Use only years, not months, when referring to spans of time in your work history. This makes it quicker for the reader to grasp the length of time, and can eliminate the need to explain some gaps that occurred within two calendar years.

2. If your unemployment covers two calendar years or more, you need to explain the void. Consider all the things you were doing (volunteer work, school activities, internships, schooling, and travel) during that time and present them in terms that are relevant to your job objective if possible.

3. If your gap has no apparent relevance to your job objective, explain the gap honestly and with dignity. References to illness, unemployment (even if it is clearly due to a recession), and rehabilitation raise red flags in most cases, so avoid those at all cost. Speak about something else that you were doing during that time, even if it doesn't relate to your job objective. Suggested "job titles":
   - Full-time Parent
   - Home Management
   - Family Management
   - Family Financial Management
   - Independent Study
   - Personal Travel

WHAT NOT TO PUT ON A RESUME

- The word "Resume" at the top of the resume
- Fluffy rambling "objective" statements
- Salary information
- Full addresses of former employers
- Reasons for leaving jobs
- A "Personal" section, or personal statistics (except in special cases)
- Names of supervisors
- References

ACCURACY/HONESTY/STRETCHING THE TRUTH

Make sure that you can back up what you say. Keep the claims you make within the range of your own integrity. There is nothing wrong with pumping things up in your resume so that you communicate who you are and what you can do at your very best.

SOME ADDITIONAL ADVICE

1. Your resume is about your future; not your past.

2. It is not a confessional. In other words, you don't have to "tell all." Stick to what's relevant and marketable.

3. Don't write a list of job descriptions. Write achievements!

4. Promote only skills you enjoy using. Never write about things you don't want to repeat.

5. Be honest. You can be creative, but don't lie.

Your name
Mailing address
City, state, and zip
Telephone number(s)
Email address

Today's date

Your addressee's name
Professional title
Organization name
Mailing address
City, state and zip

Dear Mr. (or Ms.) last name,

Start your letter with a grabber—a statement that establishes a connection with your reader, a probing question, or a quotable quote. Briefly say what job you are applying for.

The mid-section of your letter should be one or two short paragraphs that make relevant points about your qualifications. You should not summarize your resume! You may incorporate a column or bullet point format here.

Your last paragraph should initiate action by explaining what you will do next (e.g., call the employer) or instigate the reader to contact you to set up an interview. Close by saying "thank you."

Sincerely yours,

Your handwritten signature

Your name (typed)

Enclosure: resume

Your Name
Address
Telephone #

Date

Dear _____,

I am pleased to submit this resume as application for the _____ position available with your company.

Since graduating from the _____ course at (the college name), I have continued to expand my skills and am currently preparing for the _____ certification exam.

I strive to perform to the best of my ability and my work ethic is based on being a conscientious, honest, and reliable employee. I believe that the training I have received as well as my compassion for the patient will enable me to become a productive team member with your company.

I truly enjoy helping people. This is one of the greatest assets I can bring to your company. This passion is reflected in my performance and contributes greatly to my success as well as the quality of care received by my patients.

Thank you for your time and consideration.

Respectfully,

[Your Name]
[Street Address], [City, ST ZIP Code]
[phone]
[e-mail]

Objective	*Medical Assistant/Technologist position for a private practice.*

Professional Experience	**Patient Service Technician/Unit Clerk** OAK TREE COMMUNITY HOSPITAL, Coronary Care Unit, Columbus, Indiana • Order lab work and x-rays • Prioritize patient daily care according to acuity and scheduled patient procedures • Assist patients with A.M. care, take vital signs, prep for procedures, draw blood, and obtain specimens • Maintain and set up patient rooms • Perform preventive maintenance on emergency equipment • Assist with patient and family education • Assist R.N. with sterile and non-sterile dressing changes • Perform EKGs • Trained in Phlebotomy • Utilize PC to enter and retrieve patient data • Answer multi-line phone, operate fax and copy machine **Office Assistant,** (6-month part-time position) GARTH FORT, M.D., Columbus, Indiana • Answered phone, scheduled patients • Greeted patients • Updated patient charts

---

Education	In-house training programs, *Oak Tree Community Hospital* EKG, 1993 Phlebotomy, 1993 Tech Class, 1992 Unit Clerk Class, 1990 Nursing Assistant Class, 1989 CPR Certified, since 1989 *Elm Tree Community College* Computer training: WordPerfect I, Certificate 1995 *Maple Grove State University* Major: Pre-Veterinarian, 1989–1990

POWER WORDS

Accomplish	Delegate	Innovate	Publish
Achieve	Demonstrate	Inspect	Qualify
Act	Design	Install	Raise
Adapt	Detail	Institute	Recommend
Administer	Determine	Instruct	Reconcile
Advertise	Develop	Integrate	Record
Advise	Devise	Interpret	Recruit
Aid	Direct	Interview	Rectify
Analyze	Distribute	Introduce	Redesign
Apply	Draft	Invent	Reduce
Approach	Edit	Investigate	Regulate
Approve	Employ	Lead	Relate
Arrange	Encourage	Maintain	Renew
Assemble	Enlarge	Manage	Report
Assess	Enlist	Manipulate	Represent
Assign	Establish	Market	Reorganize
Assist	Estimate	Mediate	Research
Attain	Evaluate	Moderate	Resolve
Budget	Examine	Modify	Review
Build	Exchange	Monitor	Revise
Calculate	Execute	Motivate	Scan
Catalogue	Exhibit	Negotiate	Schedule
Chair	Expand	Obtain	Screen
Clarify	Expedite	Operate	Select
Collaborate	Facilitate	Order	Sell
Communicate	Familiarize	Organize	Serve
Compare	Forecast	Originate	Settle
Compile	Formulate	Oversee	Solve
Complete	Generate	Perceive	Speak
Conceive	Govern	Perform	Staff
Conciliate	Guide	Persuade	Standardize
Conduct	Handle	Plan	Stimulate
Consult	Head	Prepare	Stimulate
Contract	Hire	Present	Summarize
Control	Identify	Preside	Supervise
Cooperate	Implement	Process	Support
Coordinate	Improve	Produce	Survey
Correct	Increase	Program	Synthesize
Counsel	Index	Promote	Systematize
Create	Influence	Propose	Teach
Decide	Inform	Provide	Train

The EKG Technician Program

THE INTERVIEW

YOU HAVE 5 MINUTES

That's why first impressions—being on time, being dressed appropriately and being prepared—are critical. If you make a bad first impression, it's going to be a lot harder for you to convince someone to hire you. The interview is the most important aspect of any job hunt. The impression you make on an employer will likely be the reason you get a job offer or not.

As mentioned previously, preparation is the key to any interview. The following guidelines will assist you in presenting a positive first impression:

1. **Look Sharp**

   Before the interview, select your outfit. Depending on the industry and position, get out your best duds and check them over for spots and wrinkles.

2. **Be on Time.**

   Never arrive late to an interview. Allow extra time to arrive early in the vicinity, allowing for factors like getting lost. Enter the building 10 to 15 minutes before the interview.

3. **Do Your Research.**

   Research the company before the interview. The more you know about the company and what it stands for, the better chance you have of selling yourself.

4. **Be Prepared.**

   Bring along a folder containing extra copies of your resume, a copy of your references and paper to take notes. You should also have questions prepared to ask at the end of the interview.

5. **Show Enthusiasm.**

   A firm handshake and plenty of eye contact demonstrate confidence.

6. **Listen.**

   One of the most neglected interviewing skills is *listening*.

7. **Answer the Question Asked.**

   Candidates often don't think about whether or not they actually are answering the questions asked by their interviewers. Make sure you understand what is being asked, and get further clarification if you are unsure.

8. **Give Specific Examples.**

   One specific example of your background is worth 50 vague stories. Prepare your stories before the interview. Give examples that highlight your successes and uniqueness.

9. **Ask Questions.**

   Many interviewees don't ask questions and miss the opportunity to find out valuable information. Your questions indicate your interest in the company or job.

10. **Follow Up.**

    Whether it's through email or regular mail, *the follow-up* is one more chance to remind the interviewer of all the valuable traits you bring to the job and company. You don't want to miss this last chance to market yourself.

INTERVIEWING SKILLS

Sell It to Me, Don't Tell It to Me

Interviews are the time to sell what you have accomplished, not simply to tell what you've done. Be prepared to give examples of your accomplishments to back up you statements. An example of this is: "In my current position I suggested a change in the scheduling which allowed greater utilization of our employees and reduced turn-around-time for our customers by 20%."

This is why it is vital that you practice your responses.

- Think of what questions the interviewer may ask and practice your answers. This will allow you to make sure that your answers are clear and concise and not long winded.
- Practice will also help to reduce some of your anxiety and increase your confidence level.
- Before the interview, think of your five best strengths. What makes them strengths? Think of examples in your past performance that provides proof of these strengths and what is the best way to convey this information to the person interviewing you.
- Every interview concludes with the interviewer asking if you have any questions. The worst thing to say is that you have no questions. Again be prepared. During your research of the company did any questions arise? Did any of the statements made by the person interviewing you, provide any questions? For example; during your research you learned that the company would

be expanding their out patient facilities. This would provide an excellent opportunity to show your knowledge and interest in the future growth of the company by inquiring about this expansion.

- Never ask about benefits or salary during the interview process. The time for these questions is when the position has been offered to you.

COMMON INTERVIEW QUESTIONS

1. What are your strengths, assets, and things you do well and like about yourself?

2. What are your shortcomings, weaker points and areas for improvement?

3. Why should I hire you? How can you be an asset to this company?

4. Tell me about yourself.

5. Technical questions related to specific job functions.

6. What is your ideal coworker, supervisor or job environment?

HANDLING ILLEGAL QUESTIONS

Various federal, state, and local laws regulate the questions a prospective employer can ask you, the job candidate. An employer's questions—whether on the job application, in the interview, or during the testing process—must be related to the job you're seeking. For the employer, the focus must be: "What do I need to know to decide whether this person can perform the functions of this job?"

If asked an illegal question, you have three options:

- You can answer the question.
- You can refuse to answer the question, which is well within your rights.
- You can examine the question for its intent and respond with an answer as it might apply to the job. Let's say the interviewer asks, "Who is going to take care of your children when you are at work?" You might answer, "I can meet the work schedule that this job requires."

KEEPING TRACK OF IT ALL!

If you are keeping your promise and meeting the goal you set, you will accumulate quite a bit of data. It is important that all of this information be documented to ensure that you follow up on cold calls, cold visits, interviews etc. in a timely manner. The chart below will assist you in organizing your job search and keeping tract of those important contacts.

Job applied for	Company/contact Name	Phone/fax #	Date resume submitted	Follow up dates/comments

The EKG
Technician Program

INTERVIEW FOLLOW UP

BE PERSISTENT—NOT A PEST

A thank you note or letter is a must when looking for a job. It will set you apart from the crowd as well as provide another opportunity to be front and center in the interviewer's mind.

Your thank you letter should use the same format and presentation as your resume. It should reiterate your skills and your interest in the position being offered.

THE RETURN CALL

If you don't get a return call as promised, call them and leave a message. Be prepared, professional and courteous. Try to reach the person at least once, explaining you want the information before you consider other positions because this company is your first choice. If you don't get an answer, consider it a "No." There is a fine line between being persistent and being a pest.

You may get lucky and actually reach the person when you call. If you do have such luck, use this opportunity to ask for feedback on your interview. Sometimes, not often, a person will take the time to give you advice. If this happens, be grateful and learn from the experience.

Name of person
The person's title
Name of company
Address

Date

Dear _____:

It was a pleasure to meet with you to discuss the position of _____.

I am very excited about the chance of becoming a productive member of your team. I am confident that the extensive _____ training I have already received will enable me to represent your company with integrity and skill.

During our discussion, I sensed your strong belief in providing quality service. I want to assure you of my conviction to this important task and I will strive to perform to this standard on a daily basis.

Thank you for this opportunity and I look forward to discussing the next step in the employment process soon.

Respectfully,

The EKG Technician Program

THE JOB SEARCH

WHERE DO I START?

Looking for employment is a full time job! Tough times call for tough strategies. Take the time to sit down and create a strategy including a commitment to call, mail a resume, or visit two places of employment a minimum of three days each week. Searching for a job can be discouraging and it's important that you set goals and stick with them!

- Go through the telephone book and make a list of every facility in your area that employs your qualifications
- Network with your family and friends and let everyone know you are looking for a job
- Call your references and let them know that you will be giving out their name again. No references lined up? Get some!
- Create or update your resume

COLD CALLS

If you find that your networking prospects are drying up, it may be time to think of new ways to penetrate the job market. The cold call is a basic technique used in selling, and when done properly, it can provide new opportunities for you. If the very thought of calling a stranger and selling yourself makes you cringe, you are not alone.

- Preparing a script to read from before making the call.
- Begin with a greeting—sounding enthusiastic (but not phony) will be a plus. Introduce yourself and say what your specialty is and how many years of experience you have in your field or any training you have received
- Ask the magic question, "When can I come in for an interview?"

Not everyone you call will be interested in what you're selling. Expect rejection; two out of every three calls will not lead to new prospects. But success is the result of trying. Your career will benefit from determination and consistent effort.

When looking for employment, persistence is the key. It is hard work but once you find that dream job it will be all worth the blood, sweat and yes those tears!

HOW FLEXIBLE ARE YOU?

Today's companies are seeking employees that possess not only the knowledge to perform multiple duties but also the willingness to multitask. The rising cost of healthcare requires that job functions be diverse and multifunctional. Candidates that show an interest in learning a new skill, performing several job functions, or working various shifts are much more attractive to the potential employer than someone not willing to bend in difficult times. Often positions are offered internally to current employees. Today's candidates need to be flexible. This may require a person to take a position that is less desirable in order to be eligible to apply for the preferred position once they are an employee.

According to the Bureau of Labor Statistics . . .

"Health care will generate 3 million new wage and salary jobs between 2008 and 2016, more than any other industry."

As the largest industry in 2006, health care provided 14 million jobs—13.6 million jobs for wage and salary workers and about 438,000 jobs for the self-employed. Also, 7 of the 20 fastest growing occupations are health care related. Most workers have jobs that require less than 4 years of college education, but health diagnosing and treating practitioners are among the most educated workers.

"ONCE I HAVE THE SKILLS, WHERE CAN I USE THEM?"

Public Hospitals	Primary Care Office
Medical Clinic	Private Hospitals
Rehab Hospital	Clinical Laboratory
Independent Laboratory	Cardiology Practice
Hospital Pharmacy	Out Patient Rehab
Urgent Care Clinic	Multi-physician's Office
Home Health Care	Out Patient Laboratory
Hospice	Insurance Companies
Independent Pharmacy	Research Facility
Long-term-care Facilities	HMO's
Pharmaceutical Supply Company	Ambulatory Care Centers
Out Patient Surgery Center	Billing Company
Occupational Health	Radiology Facilities

Specialist's Office
Psychiatric Facility
VA Hospital
Pediatric Centers
Public Health Department
Chronic Care Facility
Physical Therapy Clinic
Medical Record Department

Ophthalmologist's Office
Acute Care Hospital
Cancer Centers
Birthing Center
Red Cross
Blood Banks
Sports Medicine Facility
Skilled Nursing Facility